Sometimes, multiple tests and procedures are needed to determine what is causing your pain. Back Pain Relief and Healing with Solutions Made Clear ____ ____ to you why these tests are need____ ____ ____ ____nd what some of their li

You will also learn a ____ ____ ____ ____ available to sufferer ____ ____ ____ it comes to getting re ____ ____ ____ deal with back pain. ____ ____ you with some tips you can employ ____ ____ ily life to ease the pain.

So, pick up your copy of Back Pain Relief and Healing with Solutions Made Clear so you can start your journey to living a more fulfilling and pain-free life today!

Matthew Irvine (M.ost)

been executed to present accurate, up-to-date, reliable, complete information. No warranties of any kind are declared or implied. Readers acknowledge that the author is not engaged in the rendering of legal, financial, medical, or professional advice. The content within this book has been derived from various sources. Please consult a licensed professional before attempting any techniques outlined in this book.

By reading this document, the reader agrees that under no circumstances is the author responsible for any losses, direct or indirect, that are incurred as a result of the use of the information contained within this document, including, but not limited to, errors, omissions, or inaccuracies.

Table of Contents

Back Pain Relief and Healing With Solutions Made Clear!

Content

Book Description

Tired of living in pain? Are complaints of back pain being ignored because you just don't know and can't seem to find out what is causing it?

The first step to dealing with pain is understanding what is causing it. The anatomy of the human back is extensive and complicated. How well do you know your back?

While your spine is the major collection of bones in your back, there are also discs, joints, nerves, muscles, and ligaments. Any or several could be the cause of your pain.

Back Pain Relief and Healing with Solutions Made Clear will help you understand your back and give you a clearer understanding of what may be at the root of your pain. If you are better able to understand what is causing your pain, you can better explain it to your Medical Practitioner.

When your Medical Practitioner has a better understanding of the pain you are experiencing and what may be causing it, they will be better able to select which testing methods and procedures are most likely to be the cause of the pain, thus helping to select which treatment approach would be best for your symptoms.

Back Pain Relief and Healing With Solutions Made Clear!

Content

Book Description

Tired of living in pain? Are complaints of back pain being ignored because you just don't know and can't seem to find out what is causing it?

The first step to dealing with pain is understanding what is causing it. The anatomy of the human back is extensive and complicated. How well do you know your back?

While your spine is the major collection of bones in your back, there are also discs, joints, nerves, muscles, and ligaments. Any or several could be the cause of your pain.

Back Pain Relief and Healing with Solutions Made Clear will help you understand your back and give you a clearer understanding of what may be at the root of your pain. If you are better able to understand what is causing your pain, you can better explain it to your Medical Practitioner.

When your Medical Practitioner has a better understanding of the pain you are experiencing and what may be causing it, they will be better able to select which testing methods and procedures are most likely to be the cause of the pain, thus helping to select which treatment approach would be best for your symptoms.

2

Chapter 5:

Chapter 6:

References

Introduction

Back pain is a very common ailment accounting for one of the main reasons for absence from work and seeking medical advice. Back pain can exist for a variety of reasons and is more likely to occur as we age. The human back is a complex mechanism consisting of muscles, ligaments, tendons, discs, and bones. All of these individual parts work together to allow us to move, but when one part becomes damaged, it affects the entire mechanism and leads to back pain (McIntosh, 2017).

Symptoms of Back Problems

Pain is the most common symptom of back issues. The only problem is it can occur anywhere in the back, neck, buttocks, and even down your legs. If it is nerve damage originating in the back, the pain can occur anywhere in the body. This is one of the reasons why diagnosing the issue is often difficult. Pain will often go away with rest and time. However, there are times you should go see a Medical Practitioner (McIntosh, 2017).

When to See a Medical Practitioner
According to McIntosh (2017), you should see a Medical Practitioner if any of the following accompany your back pain:

- **Weight loss**
- **Fever**
- **Persistent back pain, where lying down or resting does not help**
- **Pain down the legs**
- **Urinary incontinence**
- **Fecal incontinence, or loss of control over bowel movements**
- **Numbness around the genitals**
- **Numbness around the anus**
- **Numbness around the buttocks**

Chapter 1: Structure and Function of the Spine

In order to understand your back pain, you must first understand your back. Your spine or backbone is your body's main support structure. It consists of many individual parts working together to enable you to sit, stand, walk, bend, and twist. The following is an overview of those parts and what function each is involved in as described by The Cleveland Clinic (Spine Structure & Function, 2015).

Vertebrae

The human spine consists of thirty-three smaller bones stacked to form the spinal canal. Inside this canal are the spinal cord and nerves. The vertebrae serve two purposes, to protect the spinal cord and nerves and to allow for a range of motion. The vertebrae are able to move because of the facet joints (Spine Structure & Function, 2015).

Facet Joints

Facet joints have a slippery connective tissue known as cartilage that allows them to move against one another. This allows for the spine's flexibility and stability, allowing you to twist and turn. Your cervical joints, just below your skull, and your lumbar facet joints between your waist and hips have the most range of motion (Spine Structure & Function, 2015).

Intervertebral discs

In between each vertebra are round flat cushions with gel-like centres which act as the spine's shock absorbers. The intervertebral dics are under constant pressure, so surrounding the nucleus pulposus or gel-like centre is the annulus, a flexible outer ring. However, this ring can become damaged and tear allowing some of the gel-like substance to leak out. We will examine this issue later (Spine Structure & Function, 2015).

Spinal Cord and Nerves

Inside the spinal canal is the spinal cord which is a column of nerves that travels from your skull to your lower back. Through the neural foramen or vertebrae openings, thirty-one pairs of nerves branch out to send messages between your brain and muscles. It is our spinal cord and nerves that give us the ability to walk (Spine Structure & Function, 2015).

There are three layers, or meninges, of protective tissues around the spinal cord: the dura mater, arachnoid mater, and pia mater, with a space between each layer. The dura mater is the outermost layer and it is a tough protective coating. Then, there is a space called the epidural space, the area where a Medical Practitioner may inject a local anaesthetic for childbirth or surgery. The middle meningeal nerve of the spinal cord is the arachnoid. Between this layer and the next is a space known as the subarachnoid space. This space contains cerebrospinal fluid which Medical Practitioners can extract to test for the presence of some infections, such as meningitis. A local anaesthetic can also be injected into this area. Then, directly covering the spinal cord is the pia mater (Nall, 2019b).

If you were to take horizontal slices of the spinal cord, you would see a circular area in the middle with nerve projections extending out from it. These extend to provide feeling to different parts of the body. Key areas of a cross-section of the spinal cord would show the following. Gray matter, which is made up of nerve cell bodies, would be surrounded by the white matter which makes nerve transmissions move faster. The posterior root is a part of the nerve that branches off the spinal column and the anterior root, which branches off to the front of the spinal column. The spinal ganglion, which is a cluster of nerve bodies containing sensory neurons, and the spinal nerve, where the posterior and anterior roots come together (Nall, 2019b).

The spinal cord is involved in several key bodily functions, such as carrying signals from the brain to control movement and autonomic functions. It sends messages to the brain from the body, such as when we experience touch, physical pressure, or pain. Our motor reflexes are controlled by the spine (Nall, 2019b).

Soft Tissue
The vertebrae that make up your spine are connected and held in position by ligaments. Muscles support your back and tendons

connect these muscles to the bones. Both muscles and tendons assist you in movement. These soft tissues: ligaments, muscles, and tendons, are very important in support and movement of the spine (Spine Structure & Function, 2015).

Segments of the Spine

There are five segments to the spine, made up of thirty-three vertebrae in total. These five sections as described by Spine Structure & Function are as follows:

Cervical Spine

The cervical spine is the medical name for your neck. Your neck consists of the top seven vertebrae of your spine (C1-C7). Your cervical spine is what allows you to move your head. It has a natural C-shaped curve or lordotic curve.

Thoracic Spine

Commonly known as your middle back, your ribs are attached to your thoracic spine, forming your chest. This section naturally has a C shape called the kyphotic curve. There are twelve vertebrae in your thoracic spine, T1-T12.

Lumbar

The lumbar segment of your spine (L1-L5) makes up the lower part of your spine and is a common place for problems to occur. This is because your lower back supports your upper spine and it connects to your pelvis and supports your body weight and it bears most of the stress when you lift and carry things. The lumbar spine also has a natural lordotic curve.

Sacrum

Made from five sacral vertebrae (S1-S5), these are fused together while we are still in the womb and do not move. This triangular-shaped bone is connected to your hip bones and forms a ring that is known as the pelvic girdle.

Coccyx

These four fused vertebrae are found at the end of your spine and are commonly referred to as your tailbone. Your pelvic muscles and ligaments are attached to the coccyx (2015).

Chapter 2: Causes of Mechanical Back Pain

Acute back pain is pain that comes on suddenly and can last for up to six weeks. You may not even classify it as pain, only discomfort. This pain or discomfort can occur anywhere in your back, but it is most commonly felt in the lower back area because this area of your spine supports your body weight. While there are many reasons for lower back pain, you will usually feel it after heavy lifting, sitting for extended periods, sudden movement, or experiencing an injury or accident. It usually spasms or strains in the muscles or ligaments in the lower back that can cause acute lower back pain. Back pain can persist after an injury or surgery or can be a consequence of the bodies ageing process. Back pain is considered chronic if you experience it for three months or longer. The pain does not have to be constant, it can come and go (Low Back Pain, 2018). Often, acute back pain can lead to chronic back pain. These are some of the main causes of back pain.

Muscle and Ligament Strains

Muscle strains and sprains, particularly those in the lower back, are one of the most common causes of back pain. Your lower back or lumbar area not only supports your upper body weight, but is also directly involved in moving, bending, and twisting. A muscle strain occurs when muscle fibres are stretched too far or torn. Sprains occur when ligaments are torn from where they were attached. Both can occur suddenly or from gradual overuse. If lower back pain exists for a week or more, I suggest to make an appointment to see a Medical Practitioner. See a Medical Doctor immediately if you experience abdominal pain, fever, or loss of control over your bowels or bladder along with your back pain (Low Back Strain, n.d.).

Trapped Nerve

Also referred to as a pinched nerve, which usually occurs in your lower back. A trapped nerve in your lumbar regions can affect your back, hips, legs, ankles, and feet. If you have a trapped nerve, you will most likely feel one or several of the following: sharp pain, weakness, muscle spasms, or a loss of reflexes. Pinched nerves can happen due to injury or for what appears as no reason at all, however, there is a reason we may not be aware of. Some of the causes of a trapped nerve are herniated or bulging disc, spinal or foraminal stenosis, bone spurs, spondylolisthesis, or degenerative or rheumatoid arthritis. (Silver, 2019).

Arthritis of the Spine

According to Johns Hopkins, "Spinal arthritis is inflammation of the facet joints in the spine or sacroiliac joints between the spine and the pelvis. It may be related to wear and tear, autoimmune disorders, infection and other conditions" (Spinal Arthritis, n.d.). While there are genetic markers, age, weight and other pre-existing conditions also appear to trigger arthritis. Regardless of the cause or location, arthritis of the spine can be painful and chronic. There are two main types of arthritis, inflammatory and degenerative, both of which can affect the spine.

Inflammatory Arthritis

Rheumatoid Arthritis is an autoimmune disorder that attacks the lining of the joints. The most common area of the spine to be affected by rheumatoid arthritis is the neck, although it can occur anywhere. It may cause back pain or pain in other joints and affects women more than it does men (Spinal Arthritis, n.d.).

Degenerative Arthritis

-Osteoarthritis of the Spine

As the most common type of arthritis to affect the spine, it develops over the years through normal wear and tear as the cartilage between the joints slowly breaks down. Most pain and inflammation will be felt in the lower back when you bend or twist. Prior injuries can exacerbate the development of osteoarthritis (Spinal Arthritis, n.d.).

-Facet Joint Arthritis

When osteoarthritis affects the facet joints it is called facet disease, facet joint syndrome, or simply facet joint arthritis. Degenerative spinal discs may contribute to this type of spinal arthritis because as the discs thin, more pressure is placed on the joints, leading to more friction and damage to the cartilage (Spinal Arthritis, n.d.).

Spondyloarthritis

While not the same as rheumatoid arthritis, spondyloarthritis is a group of inflammatory diseases that affects the joints and the locations where the ligaments and tendons connect to the bones. There are several forms of spondyloarthritis:

Ankylosing spondylitis - may cause inflammation of the vertebrae and joints at the base of the spine. Extreme cases may result in a hunched back if several vertebrae fuse together.

Psoriatic arthritis - people with psoriasis may develop arthritis, although it can occur in the other order. While it usually affects small joints, it can occur in the spine as well.

Reactive arthritis - this is triggered by an infection elsewhere in the body, usually the bowels or genitals. This will usually disappear on its own with time.

Enteropathic arthritis - this form of arthritis is linked to inflammatory bowel disease (IBD) in that the IBD flare-ups usually coincide with the arthritis flare-ups. Not everyone with IBD develops arthritis and even if they do, it is not always in the spine.

Facet Lock

While we learned about facet arthritis earlier, one issue that can develop in these joints, is called a facet lock. To reiterate, they are small cartilage-like points of contact where the vertebrae of your spine meet. They control our range of mobility. The cervical (neck) facet joints and the lumbar (lower back) facet joints have the largest range of motion. If these bones get worn out, experience an injury, or develop bony spurs, they can cause a lot of pain. A locked facet joint occurs when the lower vertebrae's facet joint slips up over the one above it. This can happen on one or both sides of the vertebrae and is more likely to happen if you have weak muscles in that area. You don't have to be doing anything strenuous for this to occur, you can simply be bending or twisting. Luckily when this occurs treatment and prognosis is typically straight forward with spinal manipulation shown to be very successful in helping with facet lock symptoms (Locked Facet Joints, 2017).

Spinal Stenosis

The narrowing of the spinal canal is mostly associated with degenerative spinal disease but people can be born with it. When this occurs, there is pressure put on the spinal cord or the nerve which extends from the spine to the rest of your body. This commonly occurs in the lumbar region of your spine. This condition can cause pain when walking and you may find yourself leaning forward to relieve some of the discomfort. You may also experience pain and numbness in your legs. The most common cause of spinal stenosis is osteoarthritis, which occurs from normal wear and tear to your joints. While there is no cure for this condition, there are a lot of choices in treatments which will be discussed in detail later (Lumbar Spinal Stenosis, 2020).

Disc Problems

The intervertebral discs (disc) were introduced to you when we examined the structure of the spine. You will recall that these discs have two layers, a gel-like inside, and an elastic outer shell. These discs sit between the vertebrae of your spine and allow them to move while acting as shock absorbers. These discs can normally handle a lot of pressure but sometimes the outer ring will become weak and damaged and the inner layer can be pushed out. This is known as a protruding disc. Our discs change, as do our connective tissues as we age, it's a natural result of our spines dealing with the physical demands of our everyday life. Bulging discs, protruding of discs, and especially dehydration of our discs are all natural parts of the bodies ageing process (Services, 2020).

Spondylolisthesis

This is a condition in which one of the lower vertebrae slips forward onto one of the bones directly below it. The symptoms can go from mild to having difficulty performing everyday tasks. Spondylolisthesis can be caused by a variety of factors based on age, hereditary, or lifestyle. A birth defect or injury can result in a child having this condition. It can run in families, and sudden growth spurts during adolescence can contribute to it occurring. Also, playing sports that overstretch and put stress on your lower back such as when serving in tennis can be a factor in it forming (Moore, 2018).

Sacroiliac Joint Pain

The sacroiliac joint connects the sacrum at the bottom of your spine to the iliac bones of your pelvis. These joints are C or L shaped, strong and stable, and allow for little movement, however, they are susceptible to degenerative arthritis. The sacroiliac joints act as shock absorbers between your upper body and your pelvis and legs. This area of your body consists of dense muscles and ligaments which are the strongest ligaments in your body, and allow for little movement. Too much strain or overuse can cause tears in these ligaments, allowing for too much movement and resulting in pain (Hasz, 2015).

Lumbar Radiculopathy (Sciatica)

This condition causes pain that is associated with the compression or inflammation of a spinal nerve. While the layperson will often refer to this pain as sciatica, this is not always the correct name. The particular nerve that is being compressed or inflamed will determine the part of your lower body that is affected as the pain will follow the nerve. For example, if a nerve at the L4-5 or the L5-S1 level is affected, it is usually coming from your sciatic nerve and thus the pain will be down the back of your leg to your calf or foot as these are the nerves L4-5 and L5-S1 that supply these areas. Compression of higher lumbar nerves such as L2-3 will result in pain radiating down the front of the thigh and shin. The radicular symptoms may also come with numbness, weakness, muscle pain, and loss of reflexes. Although the pain originates in the roots of the nerves in the lumbar region of your spine, the pain can actually feel worse in your legs than in your back due to the nerves being compressed supplying this area of the body with sensation and power. Changing your standing position, walking or sitting on a soft pillow are simply tools which can usually help alleviate some of the pain felt (Ben-Yishay, 2012).

Piriformis Syndrome

The pain associated with piriformis syndrome is very similar to that associated with sciatica only it does not originate within a lumbar nerve. The piriformis is a small muscle located in the buttock region, behind the gluteus maximus, and near the sciatic nerve. This muscle starts at the lower spine and connects to each femur (thighbone). It is involved with the rotation of your hips and turning your leg and foot outwards. While it runs diagonally, your sciatic nerve runs vertically under it. This muscle can spasm, causing pain in the buttock, as well as irritating the nearby sciatic nerve, causing pain, numbness, and tingling along the back of the leg and into the foot. The exact causes of piriformis syndrome are unknown but some causes are believed to be as follows. The muscle spasms due to irritation of the muscle itself, or from the nearby sacroiliac joint, or hip. Another cause is believed to be the tightening or swelling of the muscle due to injury or spasm (Revord, 2012).

Pregnancy-Related Back Pain
Back pain is a part of pregnancy for most women simply due to the changes in their bodies. Most pregnancy related back pain occurs at the sacroiliac joint, where the pelvis meets the spine. There are likely reasons for this pain, the first being weight gain. Most women will gain between 25-35 pounds during their pregnancy and your lower spine is going to have to support that extra weight. The weight of the baby and uterus will put pressure on the nerves of the pelvis and back. Because your centre of gravity has changed, your posture will change without you noticing. This will put pressure on different parts of your spine. The hormone relaxin is released in your body during pregnancy. The purpose of this hormone is to prepare your body for childbirth by relaxing the ligaments and joints of the pelvic area. However, relaxin can also cause the ligaments that support the spine to relax causing instability and pain. The rectus abdominis muscles that run from the rib cage to the pelvic bone may separate as the uterus expands, causing back pain. Finally, emotional stress in relation to pregnancy can cause muscle tension in your back, which can lead to back spasms or pain (Dunken, 2010).

Trigger Points

Trigger points (TrP) are small knots in muscles that feels tight and compacted when compared to the muscles around them. The area can be tender and stiff and it affects your range of motion in that area. As the muscle tightens, it can cut off its own blood supply, causing further tenderness, pain, muscle spasms, and tightness. Trigger points can form all over your body. Trigger points can cause referred pain, which means the pain can travel across the whole area where the trigger point resides. For example, a trigger point in one shoulder can cause pain across your entire upper back. Almost everyone has trigger points but not all trigger points cause pain. Latent trigger points can reduce your range of motion but will only cause pain when compressed. Active trigger points can be painful even when resting. Stress, poor posture, or sleeping in an awkward position can cause latent trigger points to become active. Perhaps the most common trigger point on the human body is in the trapezius muscle which runs from the base of your neck across your shoulder and back. When we experience stress, this is the muscle that tenses up the most. It also bears a lot of pressure from handbags, briefcases, book bags, etc. It is also susceptible to whiplash. When many trigger points exist together, it is referred to as myofascial syndrome (Richeimer et al., 2019).

Chapter 3: Diagnostic Practices and Procedures

Medical diagnostic procedures can only diagnose so much, and each has an area of specialisation. According to Zinovy Meyler (2020), all Medical Practitioners should perform the following routine practices before determining whether or not further testing and or consultation is necessary:

Review the patient's past history and current symptoms. This is done by asking specific questions such as when the pain began, where it is located, other symptoms, description of the pain, and what activities or treatments ease or worsen the pain. A thorough review of past medical records is a must.

Physical examination involving several components. A visual inspection of the area and overall posture. The Medical Practitioner should put their hands on the area to check for muscle spasms and tender spots. Your range of motion should be tested to assess the mobility and alignment of the joints in the area. Finally, if nerve impingement is suspected a neurological examination will be done to test your muscle strength, skin sensation and muscles reflexes, to the area that suspected nerve impingement supplies.

A physical examination is very important because other conditions such as joint and hip issues can appear to be coming from the back. If the initial treatment, such as hands on manual therapy, ice/heat, medications, ergonomic and activity changes, is not successful or there are underlying conditions, your Medical Practitioner may want to send you for further testing.

Non-Invasive
Non-invasive simply means the testing and medical instruments stay outside the body. There is no cutting or making contact with the tissues and bones under the skin.

X rays:
The oldest electromagnetic imaging, the x-ray is the fasted and easiest way to find any problems with the bones in your spine. An x-ray will help determine any fractures or degenerative changes, such as osteoarthritis which can cause back pain. If spinal instability is suspected, flexion and extension x-rays may be ordered. This is simply the x-raying of your spine while you move your back to different positions. Soft tissue, however, cannot absorb the rays given off by the x-ray machine, therefore an x-ray is only good for determining the source of your pain if it is

located in or caused by the bones of your spine. If this is not the cause, you will have to proceed to an MRI scan (Meyler, 2020).

MRI Scans:

MRI scans provide a three-dimensional anatomical view of the bones, discs, and nerves of the spine. These scans can be key in distinguishing between acute problems and chronic conditions. MRI scans can be further enhanced with the use of a dye that can be injected through an intravenous line before or during the test itself. MRI scans are useful in diagnosing neurological symptoms for patients. Meyler, 2020).

CT Scans:

A CT scan uses radiation and a computer to create a series of cross-section images of your musculoskeletal system which is made up of muscles, bones, joints, and ligaments. These are sometimes performed with the aid of a contrasting dye as well to get a better view of the soft muscle tissue, especially if an MRI is not a viable option. CT scans can produce slice-like images of organs, bones, muscles, or fat allowing Medical Practitioners to closely examine these without having to do any invasive procedures. Where a traditional x-ray is unidirectional, a CT scan sends the x-ray beam in a circle around your body allowing for a multidirectional image to be produced on the computer screen. CT scans are best for diagnosing bone and muscle damage, tumours, infections, blood clots, or internal bleeding (Diagnosing Muscle and, 2019).

Ultrasound

An ultrasound uses sound waves and their echoes to take images of the internal structures of the body, such as in the soft tissues. Besides the traditional ultrasounds, there are now 3-D and Doppler ultrasounds available, which provide three-dimensional views and are better at illuminating blood flow throughout the body. Ultrasounds can diagnose any condition you may have affecting organs in your body, such as in your heart, bladder, kidneys, or liver. Infection or disease in these organs can manifest as back pain. Ultrasound can be effective at diagnosing possible spine disorders or tumours in newborns and infants, as they have more cartilage than bone (Spinasanta et al., 2019).

One area where ultrasound technology has proven to be useful is in image-guided diagnostic injections. Diagnostic injections try to determine the exact site of your pain by injecting numbing medication into the suspected site. The amount of immediate relief you feel indicates if the injection site was correct or not. Ultrasound technology can aid in the precision of these injection sites. Overall, ultrasounds have several appealing aspects for both patient and Medical Practitioner because there is no radiation exposure, simple to administer, widely available, inexpensive, and non-invasive. On the negative side, ultrasounds cannot provide a clear image of the bones or joints of the nearby areas (Spinasanta et al., 2019).

Bone Scan:
These are commonly used to determine the source of bone-related pain. It uses nuclear imaging to find and track bone fractures, tumours, and infections. A radioactive dye called a radiopharmaceutical is injected into the blood to assess bone metabolism. Bone metabolism refers to the ability of bones to rebuild themselves after an injury or break. Bone scans can reveal a variety of conditions including cancer, arthritis, fractures and infections in the bones. If the scan shows darker and lighter spots, it indicates that the bone is damaged and is not repairing itself. While a bone scan does subject the patient to a radioactive dye, it is no more harmful than a regular x-ray. Any radiation leaves your body through natural bodily secretions within a day

or two. Pregnant and breastfeeding women, however, should talk with their Medical Practitioner before undergoing bone scans (Crans, 2018).

SPECT Scan:

Similar to the CT scan, a SPECT scan uses a computer to create a series of cross-sectional images but these use nuclear imaging. This scan is used for the smaller, more complex bones of the spine. SPECT scan images are often used in conjunction with CT scans to get a better view of metabolic abnormalities within bones such as tumours (Meyer, 2020). A radioactive tracer is injected into the patient. This tracer then emits gamma rays, which are sent back into a gamma camera, which moves 360 degrees around the patient, allowing cross-sectional images to be shown dimensionally on the computer monitor. This scan can be used to diagnose blood flow through the heart, blockages in the arteries, degenerative brain diseases, and bone problems. Bone conditions that can be detected using a SPECT scan include hidden fractures, such as shin splints and stress fractures, cancer of the bone, and other infections. Damaged areas of the bone will be darker on a SPECT scan, while healing areas will be lighter, so the healing process can also be monitored. There is no greater risk with this scan than an x-ray and the same precautions should be taken (Garland, 2017).

DEXA Scan:

DEXA stands for dual-energy x-ray absorptiometry, meaning it sends two different energy frequency x-ray beams at the same time. DEXA scans are used to measure your bone mineral density and bone loss. One frequency beam is absorbed by the soft tissue, the other frequency by bone, then the soft tissue frequency is subtracted from the total frequency to give you your bone density. A DEXA scan is usually conducted on the lower back and hip region. This test is most frequently used to diagnose osteoporosis which aids to understand better your risk level of developing bone fractures. It can also be used to monitor the effectiveness of osteoporosis treatments in patient's (Hecht, 2019).

Electrodiagnostic Testing

Electrodiagnostic testing is used to measure the electrical activities in your nerves and muscles, specifically the speed and strength at which the electrical impulses travel between the nerves and the muscles. The test is divided into two parts:

- Nerve conduction studies (NCS) can determine nerve dysfunctions by measuring how fast it is conducting electrical signals. This is done by giving small electrical impulses to the nerve via flat electrodes attached to the skin over the nerve.

- Electromyography (EMG) is used to detect weak muscles and its interactions with nerves. This is done by inserting a needle electrode into the muscles.

A slow or weak transmission from one point to another can indicate a impinged or damaged nerve. Sciatica and carpal tunnel syndrome are two common conditions that can be diagnosed through electrodiagnostic testing (Electrodiagnostics, n.d.).

More Invasive

More invasive, or simply invasive, involves cutting open the skin or puncturing the skin with a needle to go deeper into a cavity of the body.

Lumbar Discography

A discography or discogram is an imaging test used to determine which spinal disc could be the cause of back pain. This invasive procedure should only be done for patients with persistent pain, those who have already undergone other testing methods with no success at finding the cause of their pain. A lumbar discography can be the last step before surgery or to determine if surgery will be effective. During this procedure, a radiologist will inject dye into a few select discs in the area of the patient's pain to try to determine which one may be causing the pain. With the use of an x-ray and CT monitor, the dye will allow the image to indicate if there are any tears or herniation in the discs. There will be some pain felt by the patient during this procedure, as its purpose is to provoke existing pain but it should not be any greater than what the patient normally feels (Shiel, 2020).

Nerve Conduction Test

Nerve conduction velocity (NCV) tests measure how quickly nerve signals move through your peripheral nerves in an attempt to assess any damage or dysfunction. Your peripheral nerves are located along your spinal cord and they help you control your muscles and experience feelings of sensation. A NCV test can help your Medical Practitioner determine if an injury is affecting the nerve itself or the myelin sheath, the covering around the nerve. It can also help differentiate between a nerve condition and a nerve injury that is affecting the muscles. A NCV test can help determine if you are suffering from herniated disc disease, carpal tunnel syndrome and sciatic nerve problems among others. An Electromyography is often performed with a NCV test (Connor, 2018).

Lumbar Puncture

A lumbar puncture, commonly known as a spinal tap, is a neurological procedure used to diagnose a wide variety of conditions. In this procedure, a needle is inserted between the bones of your lower back, and a sample of cerebrospinal fluid is removed for further study. While a lumbar puncture is most commonly used to test for meningitis, it is also helpful in diagnosing bacterial, viral, and fungal infections, inflammatory diseases, some cancers of the spine, or inflammation of the spinal cord. It can also be used to measure the pressure of the cerebrospinal fluid around your brain and spinal cord. (Pressman, 202).

Sacroiliac Joint Injections

The sacroiliac joints connect your spine to your pelvis and forms your lower back and buttocks region. When this joint is the cause of your pain, the pain can be felt in the immediate region, groin, abdomen, hips, buttocks, or legs. In this procedure, the Medical Practitioner will use an x-ray to guide a small needle into the joint, then inject contrasting dye to ensure the needle is in the right location. Once the correct location is confirmed, a mixture of numbing medication and anti-inflammatory cortisone will be injected. After twenty or thirty minutes, you will be asked to move to try to provoke the usual pain you feel. You will report your level of pain at the time and also keep a pain record for the next week. The amount of pain you feel, if any, will determine whether or not the sacroiliac joint is the cause of your pain or not. If you do not feel relief within ten days, you are not likely to get any and further testing will be required to determine the cause of your symptoms (Dreyfuss, 2019).

Human Leukocyte Antigen B27 (HLA-B27)

Human Leukocyte Antigen B27 (HLA-B27) is a protein located on the surface of white blood cells. Human leukocyte antigens help your immune system differentiate between healthy tissue and foreign substances that may cause infection. If you have HLA-B27 on your white blood cells, it triggers your immune system to destroy healthy cells. This can lead to autoimmune diseases or immune-mediated diseases. The presence of HLA-B27 can be detected with a blood test. This blood test may be ordered if your Medical Practitioner suspects that inflammation of the bones or joints in your spine may be the cause of your symptoms (Burke, 2018).

Chapter 4: Physical and Manual Therapy

There is a wide variety of pain management procedures, applications, and machinery that can help you cope with back pain. From hands-on to use of medical equipment and exercises you can do on your own prescribed by a Medical Practitioner.

Spinal Manipulation
Spinal manipulation is a hands-on approach to treating back pain. Commonly but not exclusively used by Chiropractors, Osteopaths, Osteopathic Physicians, and Physiotherapists. Developed to treat tension in joints it is now used to treat a wide variety of musculoskeletal symptoms including but not exclusive to lower back, neck, rib, and shoulder symptoms.

Spinal manipulation. Using their hands, the Practitioner will apply a controlled sudden force to a specific joint. This often results in popping or cracking noises coming from the joint being worked on.

Practitioners may also wish to use heat and ice therapy, electric stimulation, traction devices, to stretch the spine and ultrasound therapy for deep tissue heating to compensate their spinal manipulations. When performed by a properly trained and licensed Medical Practitioner, spinal manipulation carries little risk. There are certain individuals who should refrain from getting this type of treatment. Anyone with severe osteoporosis, are at high risk of a stroke or have spinal cancer should not receive this treatment (Morris, 2016).

Some Medical practitioners use activators when treating patients. This is a spring-loaded, handheld instrument that allows the

Practitioner to administer a quick, low-force impulses at specific points on the patient's body. There are two cited advantages to using an activator device:

- High speed. When applied to the muscles of the body, the pulse is so fast, they do not get a chance to tense up. The less tense muscles are, the more effective the manipulation will be.

- Controlled force. The force is localised, so the joint is not put in compromising positions, such as bending or twisting which is required for when doing a hands on spinal manipulation.

To date, there are no results to prove that the use of an activator provides any better results than manual manipulation. As with manual manipulation, certain patients should not undergo activator treatments. Patients should undergo an examination prior to treatment to ensure they do not have pain as a result of infection, cancer, fracture, or open wound (Minx, 2020).

Massage
Massage is recognised as a legitimate aid for lower back pain. It is now being recommended by over 50% of Medical Physicians in addition to other back pain treatments. According to Beth Mueller, "A study on massage and back pain, conducted at The Touch Research Institute at the University of Miami in 2001, found that: 'Massage lessened lower back pain, depression, and anxiety, and improved sleep. The massage therapy group also showed improved range of motion and their serotonin and dopamine levels were higher," (2002).

The benefits of massage therapy according to the American Massage Therapy Association include:

- **Improved blood circulation. This aids in the recovery of tense muscles especially useful after physical activity.**

- **Relaxes muscles. Relaxed muscles improve the range of motion and helps reduce insomnia.**

- **Increases endorphin levels. This is perhaps the biggest benefit of massage therapy. Endorphins are chemicals produced by the body that make you feel good, which is a very effective tool in managing pain (Mueller, 2002).**

Neuromuscular Massage

Neuromuscular massage therapy is seen as the most effective type of massage for lower back pain caused by soft muscle injury such as muscle strains. This form of massage therapy consists of applying alternating levels of concentrated pressure on areas of the muscle spasm. This pressure is applied manually with the fingers, knuckles, or elbows. According to Mueller, "Muscles that are in spasm will be painful to the touch. The pain is caused by ischemic muscle tissue. Ischemia signifies that the muscle is lacking proper blood flow, usually due to the muscle spasm" (2002). When the muscle does not receive the proper amount of blood, it also does not receive enough oxygen. This causes the muscle to produce lactic acid, and it is the lactic acid that makes the muscle feel sore. When muscles are massaged, the lactic acid is removed from the muscle, allowing it to receive the proper amount of oxygen and blood. This type of massage can be painful at the beginning but it should alleviate the pain. Communication between patient and therapist is important as the procedure should never be overly painful. Any soreness experienced after massage should disappear within twenty-four to thirty-eight hours (Mueller, 2002).

Massage therapy has been found to work best in combination with other medical treatments given by practitioners such spinal manipulation, acupuncture and dry cupping (Mueller, 2002).

Acupuncture and Back Pain

Acupuncture is an ancient Chinese therapy based on the idea of energetics in the body. Acupuncture consists of inserting needles through the skin at various pressure points on the body. This energy (qi in Chinese) points are called meridians and there are several qi meridians an acupuncturist may focus on for back pain. According to Adrian White, some of the acupuncture points for lower back pain are found in the back of the knees, foot, lower back, hand, hip, and stomach. For upper back pain, qi meridians are located on the head, neck, shoulders, and upper back. By stimulating these points, parts of the nervous system are stimulated to relieve pain, (2019).

It is not entirely understood how acupuncture works to relieve back pain, but these as some of the beliefs of its practitioners:

Stimulation of the nervous system. When trigger points are stimulated by the acupuncture needle, chemicals are released by the spinal cord, muscles, and brain. Some of these chemicals can be natural pain relievers.

Releases opioid like chemicals. Similar to the theory above, it is believed that acupuncture causes the body to release natural pain relieving chemicals, with similar properties to opioid pain relievers.

Releases neurotransmitters. Neurotransmitters are hormones that send messages to various nerve endings. It is believed that acupuncture may stimulate some that shut off pain.

Triggers electromagnetic impulses. These electromagnetic impulses may release endorphins that speed up the way the body handles pain.

Regardless of how it works, there is very little risk of adverse side effects from acupuncture. White also summarised studies from 2012 that interviewed 20,000 people with back pain. Of those who received acupuncture, 50% said they experienced improvements with their chronic back pain issues (2019). In the western world many Medical Practitioners use acupuncture but instead of applying the needles following the bodies meridians they are using their palpatory skills to find tender spots in muscles and applying the needles in these areas.

Dry Cupping

Cupping is an ancient therapy practiced by Chinese and Middle Eastern medical professionals for centuries. With this form of therapy, the practitioner places cups on your back, stomach, arms, legs, or other parts of your body to relieve pain. Inside the cup, there is a vacuum or suction force that pulls the skin up and increases the blood flow in that area. While there are not a lot of studies on how cupping actually helps, the general belief of how it works is that the suction draws fluid up into that area. The suction's force breaks open small blood vessels (capillaries) under the skin. The body, in turn, treats the area with the broken capillaries as an injury, sending more blood to the area to aid in the healing process. Another theory is that cupping unclogs pores and releases toxins (Cupping: Back Pain, 2020).

Unlike in ancient Chinese acupuncture, the cups are placed on the area where the pain is being experienced. By increasing the blood flow to that area, the muscles get the supply of oxygen and nutrients it needs to repair itself and ease the pain. Cupping can accurately target the joint or muscle causing the pain. Cupping can release tension in the tissues of your body, relax sore, tense muscles, and thus ease back and neck pain. Cupping it self causes certain changes to occur within the body, stimulating to heal itself. The results according to Sirfraz Nazir (2018) are:

- Promoting the flow of blood to the muscles and tissues thus aiding in preventing stagnation

- Supplying oxygen and nutrients to the cells.

- Softening tightened muscles.

- Loosening of adhesions and knots in muscles.

- Lifting connecting tissues which lines all muscles in the body.

- Opening the blockages of lymphatic nodes and easing the flow of lymph.

- Releasing and draining excess fluids and toxins like lactic acid from the tissues and cells.

- Drawing inflammation from the deeper tissues to the surface of the skin so they can heal.

Infrared Light Therapy

Infrared light therapy uses certain wavelengths of light to target sites on the body that have injuries as a treatment to relieve chronic and acute pain. Infrared light helps cells regenerate and repair themselves, improves the circulation of blood and oxygen throughout the body, aiding in the healing of deep tissues, and relieving pain. Infrared light is the heat that we feel from the sun which is able to penetrate the skin without damaging it as ultraviolet light does. Infrared light has been shown to have many health benefits from pain relief to reducing inflammation (Laguipo, 2019).

Infrared light therapy works by using technology to allow people to receive the benefits to the sun without the dangers of ultraviolet rays. The infrared light penetrates from two to seven centimetres under the skin, to reach muscles, nerves, and even bones. The light is absorbed by the photoreceptors in cells, initiating several naturally occurring cellular processes. Nitric oxide is believed to be the key to the efficiency of infrared light therapy. "Nitric oxide is a potent cell signalling molecule that helps relax the arteries, battles free radicals to reduce oxidative stress, prevents platelet clumping in the vessels, and regulates blood pressure. Hence, this molecule enhances blood circulation to deliver vital nutrients and oxygen to damaged and injured tissues in the body" (Laguipo, 2019). Infrared light therapy can be an effective way to treat lower back and neck pain caused by muscle strain and arthritis

Ultrasound Therapy

Ultrasound therapy uses sound waves (vibrations) to treat medical conditions, however, very little evidence can be provided to prove that it is beneficial to helping with back pain. Ultrasound therapy consists of placing a hand-held ultrasound machine onto the pained area as it omits sound waves, delivering heat and energy to the body to reduce pain and speed up the recovery process. The main benefit that can be shown, is improving the range of motion in the soft tissue of the spine. Therefore, it would be best used in conjunction with manual therapy such as massage and spinal mobilisation (Malanga, 2019).

Shockwave Therapy

Shockwave therapy involves applying a series of low-energy acoustic wave pulsations to an injured area, through the patient's skin with the aid of a gel medium. This has been proven through several scientific studies to be a successful treatment for a number of chronic conditions. The purpose of shockwave therapy is to kickstart the body's own healing process and many people feel a reduction in pain and increases mobility after their treatments. It is primarily used to treat musculoskeletal conditions involving connective tissues such as ligaments and tendons. While new studies are showing promising results in the use of shockwave therapy for acute pain, more research will need to be conducted before it is widely accepted in this area of pain treatment (Afshar, 2017).

Shockwave therapy is usually done once a week for three to six weeks. While it may be mildly uncomfortable, it should only last for four or five minutes. In terms of back pain, it has been shown to be effective for the relief of pain in the lumbar and cervical spine regions and chronic muscular pain. There are some unpleasant, yet manageable side effects of this therapy, such as tenderness, soreness, and swelling. However, as it is triggering your body's natural healing process, this is to be expected. It is important that you do not take painkillers to deal with this discomfort as it may slow down the process (Afshar, 2017).

TENS Machines
Transcutaneous electrical nerve stimulation (TENS) machines may not deal with the underlying condition causing your chronic back pain, it may help you deal with the pain and other symptoms. A TENS unit is a battery-operated device that uses electrodes attached near the painful area, to deliver low or high-intensity electrical impulses. While the science behind the use of electrical nerve stimulation to ease back pain is not fully understood, according to Sandra Gordon, two theories are proposed:

- On a low frequency, it stimulates larger diameter pain fibres so the brain doesn't hone in on the pain generated from smaller diameter pain fibres. Known as the gate control theory of pain.

- On a high frequency setting set on the TENS machine, a TENS unit for back pain is believed to work by releasing local neurotransmitters, such as endorphins, at nerve endings to block pain signals (2020).

Regardless of how it actually works, it should not be relied on solely. Most of the relief you will receive from a TENS unit is during use, possibly for several hours afterward. Gordon (2020) quotes Dr. Khan when informing us that there are also several things you must keep in mind while using a TENS unit:

Check with your Medical Practitioner first, especially if you have an electrical implant, you are pregnant, you have epilepsy, or any heart problems. Do not use it if you have a pacemaker.

For the most benefit, limit your sessions to ten or fifteen minutes in muscle stimulation mode. You can go up to two hours for total spine pain but any longer than that is not recommended as it may irritate the skin.

While a TENS unit may not get to the root of your problem, it may help you perform your daily routines more efficiently and comfortably.

IDD Therapy
Intervertebral Disc distraction (IDD) therapy has grown substantially over the past ten years in the quest to alleviate back and sciatica pain. While most back and sciatica pain will get better with a combination of rest and manual therapy, the biggest problem Manual therapists face is dealing with the ineffectiveness of using standard hands on procedure for lower back pain. This can be especially difficult when the problem is associated with a spinal or intervertebral disc

issue. A bulging or herniated disc can cause pain in the neck or lower back. When the disc presses against a nerve exiting the spinal column, it can cause pain to radiate down the arms or legs (radiculopathy). By combining computer science and physics with the human anatomy, IDD therapy spinal compression was born (Hazlegreaves, 2019).

IDD therapy gave Manual therapists a new way to decompress and mobilise specific spinal segments, allowing for greater success in certain treatment of lower back and neck issues. A SPINA machine is used to deliver IDD therapy, which a person is tied to via two harnesses at the spine, and the pelvis. Then a computer is used to apply a gentle pulling force, at precisely measured angles, to open up the space between the vertebrae. This takes the pressure off the affected disc. Higher pulling forces can then be increased in intervals with the lower force. This helps mobilise the joints, leading to overall increased mobility of the spine. This increased spinal mobility helps in the exchange of fluids and nutrients needed for healing process to occur (Hazlegreaves, 2019).

Postural Training
Proper posture reduces stress on your muscles and ligaments and decreases your chance of injury. Posture training can help you develop strength, balance, and flexibility. It also creates an awareness of your body and your natural posture and allows you to develop the muscles necessary to correct your posture.

Yoga
Yoga is not simply an exercise program, it is a holistic approach to health and wellness. Its aim is to unite the body, mind, and spirit to create physical and mental benefits. While there are many different types of yoga, they are all based on three main components: body posture, breathing, and meditation. All of

these components can help those suffering from back pain.

Yoga involves holding positions anywhere from ten to sixty seconds. This requires concentration and the use of certain muscle groups. As yoga focuses on body posture, the muscle groups involved are those of the back and abdomen, the same muscles that compose the muscular network of the spine. When these muscles are strengthened, back pain can be reduced or prevented. Tension on the load-carrying muscles of the back can also be relieved through the stretching and relaxation exercises of yoga as well. In certain poses, some muscles are flexed while others are stretched, leading to greater flexibility of the muscles and joints. Proper conditioning of these muscles will improve posture, balance, and proper alignment, all of which can prevent or reduce back pain. Even the basic stretching exercises of yoga can help those with back pain as it increases blood flow which allows nutrients to flow in and toxins to flow out. (Busch, 2014).

Pilates
Pilates is an exercise program developed to create an awareness of the natural alignment of the spine and to strengthen the core muscles that sport this alignment. Pilates encourages the participant to develop the following skills: improve movement efficiency and muscle control through mental focus, and awareness of proper posture, how to develop the muscles of the back and abdomen to support posture, mental focusing through proper breathing, and to lengthen, strengthen and increase the flexibility of their muscles. This focus on the spine and its muscles make Pilates an excellent exercise program to prevent and relieve back pain (Glosten, 2003).

Those with back pain caused by excessive movement or degeneration of disc and joints would most benefit from Pilates. With improved posture, there will be less pressure and wear and tear on the joints and discs of the entire spine. By strengthening and increasing the durability of the muscles of the hip and shoulder girdle, Pilates helps prevent unnecessary torque on the vertebral column (Glosten, 2003). Perhaps the most beneficial principles of the Pilates program is the awareness of proper posture, movement, and breathing it creates in the individual, allowing them to prevent and improve back pain through everyday activities.

Tai Chi

Tai Chi is a healing exercise program emphasising slow and soft movements and a sense of inner calmness and tranquillity. While it may look similar to yoga, it encompasses a greater degree of movement. Tai Chi provides all the benefits of low-impact exercises while focusing on improved posture, balance, and alignment. The breathing involved promotes blood flow and a relaxed body. The meditative state of mind decreases stress and anxiety which can help back pain caused by psychological and emotional factors (Humphreys, 2004).

Chapter 5: Tips to Living with Back Pain

There are many things that we do on a daily basis without giving much thought to the wear and tear we can be unnecessarily putting on our muscles, ligaments, and joints, especially those of our back. Our back is very important as it is our weight-bearing centre of gravity and we need to take care of it. These are some of the little things we can do that will make a big difference to those who are experiencing back pain and for those who are not, it could prevent you from experiencing it in the future.

Getting Out of Bed

What is the first thing we do every morning? We wake up and get out of bed. For some, this simple action most of us take for granted can be the beginning of a very painful day. It is important that we get out of bed without causing stress to our back and, the most important thing to remember is to not twist our back. Start by lying on your back and taking a few deep breaths while gently elongating your body. Bend your knees so that your feet are flat on the bed. Now, roll your entire body to the side, towards the outside of the bed, at the same time. Use both of your hands to push yourself into a sitting position. In the sitting position, make sure your weight is evenly distributed and sit up straight, arching your back. Put one foot in front of the other and keeping bended knees, bend forward from the hip, keeping your back straight. Press your feet down into the floor and straighten both legs at the same time as you rise. Bring your back foot forward to meet the front (2020). Now, you are ready to conquer the day!

Putting on Your Shoes
Use a shoehorn. Every day, we put shoes on and most of us bend at the waist to do so. Bending at the knees to complete this task is often awkward. A shoehorn allows you to put your shoes on with just a slight bend of the knees. There are many lengths and sizes of shoe horns which can be purchased to suit your requirements.

Making Your Bed and Doing Laundry
Both of these activities often require a lot of bending, but bending should be done at the knees and not the waist. When making your bed, bend your knees and use your arms to support your weight, and keep your balance as you straighten and tuck your sheets and blankets in. The same technique should be used when taking clothes out of the washing or drying machines. Use your knees for

bending and your forearms to bear your weight. If using a clothesline to dry your clothing, place the basket directly in front of your feet and bend at the knee to retrieve the items. Make sure your line is not too high, causing you to overextend to reach it (Mitchell, 2019).

Vacuuming and Mowing Your Lawn
Keep the vacuum or mower close to your body and bend slightly at the knee as you walk forward. Keep your upper body straight, this will put you in a partial lunge not only protecting your back but strengthening it as well. Use long sweeps from one end of the area to the opposite to minimise turning and jarring of your joints (Mitchell, 2019).

Food Shopping
While in the food shopping store, always try to use a wheeled cart so as to not be carrying a basket. Ask for assistance when reaching for high objects and bend at the knees when able to search lower shelfs. When carrying the bags into your house, make as many trips as possible to lighten your load. It is often tempting to load up and make only one trip but this is putting unnecessary strain on your back. If you must carry a heavy item, hold it close to your chest, supporting it with your abdomen and thigh muscles. Make sure the walk from your car to your house is free of obstacles as unexpected falls can hurt more than just your back (Mitchell, 2019).

Gardening
Gardening can be a very taxing activity for anyone as it involves a lot of bending, kneeling, and lifting. Pacing yourself is key. Take a lot of breaks and do a lot of stretching. Avoid being bent or stooped for long periods of time. Your muscles and joints need to be active, they do not like to be in the same position for extended periods. If you are potting plants and you are able to bring them up to your level, this is best. If not, kneel down in front of them, do not bend or stoop. If you need to move a heavy plant, rest it against

your thighs and lunge to the side, and shift your weight from one leg to the other. This way your larger thigh muscles are supporting the weight instead of your back. Try not to twist as you move to the side, remain facing forward. If you are planting directly in the ground, use knee pads or a cushion to protect your knee joints. Placing a hand on the ground or on your thigh will help you keep your balance. Always try to keep your upper back straight and bend from your hips (Mitchell, 2019).

Washing Dishes, Cooking, Ironing

These household chores involve a lot of standing and they give you the perfect opportunity to work on strengthening your core muscles. These muscles in your abdomen, back, and sides, work together to support your spine. Take a deep breath and draw your belly button in towards your spine. Then, tuck your tailbone beneath you and contract your gluts. Do this repeatedly while completing your chores (Mitchell, 2019).

Interacting with Children

When playing with your children, movement is key. You may be sitting on the floor, kneeling, or lying down. Change positions frequently, get up, and move around even if it is just to pick up a toy. Try to remain cognisant of your posture, no matter what position you are in. When picking up your child, take the time to think about doing it properly. Bend your back, knees, and hips, slightly forward and press them tight to your body. Use your leg muscles to return to a standing position, keeping your back straight. Try not to twist or turn while picking your children up (Mitchell, 2019).

Using a Mobile Phone

Millions of people use one every day without giving it a second thought. They are such small devices, who would stop to think that using a cell phone could be detrimental to your back? Due to the way we tilt our heads forward and down when using them, we are doubling, possibly tripling the weight of our head, and that weight is supported by our neck. The way we use cell phones and tablets is more than just a pain in the neck! It is also leading to pain in the shoulders, arms, and the upper mid back. The average human head weighs between ten and twelve pounds and that weight is supported by the neck muscles, tendons, and ligaments during movement and also when static. When we tilt our heads forward, we are engaging the use of our intervertebral discs that help absorb and distribute the forces exerted on our necks (Ammerman, 2019).

Joshua Ammerman (2019), has interestingly referred to computerised models that have come up with the following information on the strain placed on our necks when we tilt our heads forward: 15 degrees equates to the head weighing 27 pounds of strain, 30 degrees = 40 pounds, 45 degrees = 49 pounds, and 60 degrees = 60 pounds of strain. The average person has their head tilted forward two to four hours per day, teenagers even more, and as you tilt your head, your shoulders curve forward. This excess strain and wear and tear on the neck, shoulders, and upper back can lead to spinal degeneration. To reduce the risk of spinal degeneration, there are several things we can do. For example we can use a computer or laptop for extended internet browsing, not a tablet or cell phone. Try to raise your phone up to eye level when using it instead of tilting your head down.

Acute Back Pain

Lower back pain can come and go. When it comes, it can be sudden and debilitating. There are some simple things you can do at home to deal with the pain caused by acute back injuries. If you have tweaked your back, for the first 24 to 48 hours, try applying ice. Using preferably a cold pack, wrap it in a cloth, and apply to your lower back for no more than ten minutes. Reapply as often as needed, making sure to remove for at least ten minutes before reapplying. After one or two days, you can replace the cold compound with heat. In the same fashion, make sure the heat is wrapped, to prevent injury to the skin. Apply in ten-minute sessions, same as the ice. During the first 48 hours, it is vital to rest, to allow your back to start the healing process (Nall, 2019).

Movement is Key

Unless you are experiencing acute back pain and you are going through the rest/ice/heat regime, movement is key to a healthy back. Our bodies were meant to move and many of the key functions of our bodies need movement to work efficiently. One of the components of our bodies that need movement is the discs of our spine. Discs receive their nutrients via fluid. Acting like a sponge, a healthy disc will absorb fluid then squeeze out the water, distributing the nutrients to the disc. This Fluid exchange also reduces swelling in surrounding soft tissue, which naturally occurs when a disc is damaged. When there is a lack of exercise swelling increases around the disc further damaging the disc as it becomes malnourished. Movement increases flexibility and mobility in ligaments and tendons which surround the spine lessening the chance of tearing under stress. Any sort of movement helps to strengthen, stretch, and repairs muscles that support the back (Hochschuler, 2004).

Walking can be a beneficial form of low-impact exercise for people with ongoing or recurring lower back pain. Many people with low back pain are not able to take part in other aerobic exercises as it puts too much stress on an already injured area. Exercise walking, however, is a low-impact aerobic exercise that will not aggravate the lower back. Walking strengthens the muscles of the feet, legs, hips, and torso. It increases the spine's stability and works the muscles that keep the body upright. Walking nourishes the spinal structures by increasing circulation which pumps nutrients into soft tissue and drains toxins. Along with regular stretching, walking allows for a greater range of motion. Walking helps to prevent bone density loss which can help prevent osteoporosis and aid in building bone strength, which in turn can reduce osteoporosis symptoms in patients. Walking can help maintain a healthy weight which will help reduce stress on our weight-bearing spine. Before starting to walk, you should do some gentle stretching to prepare the joints and muscles for the increased range of motion they will be experiencing. Then, walk slowly for about five minutes to warm the muscles up before stretching some more. Start out with a five-minute walk and work up to thirty minutes at least three to four times a week (Forcum & Hyde, 2004).

Lumbar Support Belts

When designed well, a back support belt can relieve back pain caused by muscle strain, spasms and disc problems. By constraining muscles and ligaments, support belts can encourage better posture and give extra support and stability when lifting. Restricting the motion of discs, joints, and muscles support belts can decrease the pressure exerted on disc and facet joints as you bend forward and backwards. This restriction in bending also leads to developing proper lifting techniques. You are not able to bend far enough at the waist, therefore you rely on bending your knees, which is the proper way to lift, yet we seldom do it because it expends more energy to do so. Compression in the form of a belt can help manage and reduce inflammation as well as perform warmth for increased circulation (Ornstein, n.d.).

Taping

Kinesiology (Kinesio) tape has many benefits including providing support, lessening pain, and reducing inflammation. Kinesio tape was formulated to mimic your skin, it is made from a blend of cotton and nylon and is very stretchy, allowing you to use your full range of motion. It also uses a medical-grade adhesive so that you do not have to worry about it getting wet or sweaty. It can stay on for three to five days even while you take part in all your regular daily life activities. Kinesio tape lifts your skin by recoiling slightly after application, creating a space between your skin and the tissue underneath, (Stanborough, 2019).

According to Rebecca Stanborough, studies have shown that kinesiology tape can create space in joints, particularly in the knee and shoulder joints. When space is increased, it helps reduce joint irritation, thus decreasing pain. It may also help increase blood flow in the skin and may improve the circulation of lymphatic fluid. These fluids are involved in the body's swelling and fluid buildup. It is proposed that when this tape recoils and creates a space between your skin and the tissues underneath, the pressure gradient changes to enhance lymphatic fluid flow. This increase in lymphatic fluid flow may also help speed up the healing of bruises. (2019).

Manual Therapists frequently use kinesiology tape to treat trigger points. When placed over tense and knotted muscles the skin lifts the area is decompressed and tension in the trigger point decreases. Kinesio Tape is used to reduce pain and swelling, not alone but in conjunction with manual therapy. It can be used to give extra support to injured or weakened muscles and joints. It may even help retrain muscles and has been used with stroke patients who are learning to walk. Do not use Kinesio tape over open wounds, if you suffer from deep vein thrombosis, have had a lymph node removed, an allergy to adhesives, or have fragile skin (Stanborough, 2019).

Posture
Good posture is a must for keeping the structures of the back and spine healthy. Your posture plays a critical role in the frequency and intensity of incidents of back and neck pain. If you spend hours sitting or standing

during the day, proper posture is of extreme importance. Over time, poor posture can change the anatomical characteristics of the spine, possibly leading to constricted blood vessels and nerves and problems with muscles, discs, and joints. This in turn can cause lower back and neck pain, headaches, fatigue. Having good posture means all of your body parts are aligned, balanced, and supported (Schubbe, 2004).

Identifying Good Posture

When standing, there should be a straight line from the earlobe, through the shoulder, hips, knee to the middle of the ankle. However, we spend very little time standing straight but instead move frequently throughout the day to bend, sit, stoop, or lay down. By keeping a good posture, we can perform all these actions efficiently without having to think much about it. It is important to remember that our spines are made for moving, so it is important to get up and move around during the day. Stand and stretch regularly during the day to help prevent our muscles, ligaments, and joints from becoming overly stiff (Schubbe, 2004).

The best way to improve your posture is to access what you are doing wrong. Throughout the day with the aid of a mirror, look at how you stand, sit, bend and carry things, etc. Make a mental note of your posture so that you can identify the times and positions when you had poor posture. According to Schubbe (2004), the following are examples of things we do that contribute to poor posture:

- Slouching with shoulders pulled forward.

- Standing or sitting with too large of an inward curve in the lower back.

- Carrying something heavy on one side of our body.

- **Cradling a phone between our shoulder and neck.**

- **Wearing high-heeled shoes or clothing that is too tight.**

- **Sleeping with a mattress or pillow that does not provide proper support.**

There are things we can do to help correct these mistakes we make on a daily basis. It may be uncomfortable and feel foreign at first, but with persistence, they will come to you naturally, (Schubbe, 2004).

Standing Posture
With the focus on too much sitting in today's world, we are now trying to incorporate more moving and even standing into our daily activities. Most experts recommend we get 20 minutes of standing every hour, however, in our work efficiency culture, we still want to continue to be productive as we stand. Thus, came the invention of the sit-stand desk. These desks allow you to transition easily from sitting to standing without compromising your workstation. If you don't have a sit-to-stand workstation, you can still stand for the good of your spine, while working. You could work while standing at a counter or high table, (Malanga, 2019)

To simply get up and stand is not enough. You need to make sure you are standing efficiently so that you do not put undue pressure on your spine and other joints. According to John Schubbe, the proper standing posture is as follows:

- **Stand with most of your weight on the balls of your feet, not on the heels.**

- **Feet should be shoulder width apart.**

- **Arms should hang naturally down the sides of your body.**

- **Do not lock your knees.**

- **Tuck your chin in to keep head level.**

- **Head should be straight with your spine, not pushed forward.**

- **Straight and tall, with shoulders squared.**

- **Shift weight from foot to foot or rock back and forth from toes to heels if you must stand for a long period of time.**

- **Stand against a wall with buttocks and shoulders touching the wall. The back of your head should be touching as well, if not you carry your head too far forward (2004).**

Walking Posture

Walking is a low-impact exercise that can have many benefits for those with back pain. You should always maintain proper form when walking to protect your back and prevent injury.

Head and shoulders. Keep your head up and centred between your shoulders. Your eyes should be focused straight ahead. Keep your shoulders straight, yet relaxed, never slouch forward.

Hips. Your hips should guide your stride and should feel natural. Do not try to lengthen or shorten your stride, so use what comes naturally.

Arms and hands. Your arms should be close to your body and elbows at a 90-degree angle. Your arms should swing, comfortably from front to back in pace with the stride of the opposite leg. Your hands should be relaxed, slightly cupped, palms inward, and thumbs on top.

Feet. You should always land lightly on your heel and midfoot, rolling forward to the balls of your feet, then pushing off with your toes, (Forcum & Hyde, 2004).

Driving Posture

Vehicles have had so many advances over the years and many have seats with height, tilt, lumbar support, heating, etc. Yet, many of us do not take the time to adjust our seats so that they give us the best support to prevent injury, especially if we share the driving with other people. We are too busy, we just get in the car, maybe adjust the distance between our seat and the throttle, then we are on our way!

Driving is different from regular sitting because your body is constantly subjected to different forces: acceleration and deceleration, side to side swaying, and up-down vibrations. Some of these forces can be gentle, some quite jarring! Your feet, normally used to stabilise and support your body are also in use. Commonly your right foot is on the accelerator pedal while your left foot is poised ready to break, or in the case of a standard transmission, it is being used on the clutch pedal. These factors, combined with the design of cars and car seats, can lead to back problems in some individuals (Hedge, 2019a).

Hedge reported the following findings: "A comparison of drivers in the USA and in Sweden found that in each country 50% of those questioned reported low back pain...long term vibration exposure from driving was among the highest risk factors for neck, back and low back problems...The Swedish study of over 1,000 salespeople found significantly increased risks of neck and low back pain among those who drove long distances and spent a large proportion of time each day in their car" (2019).

Based on scientific journals and text, automotive engineering reports, and the

National Library of Medicine, the following optimal car seat was developed. According to Hedge, "the optimal car seat should have:

- **Adjustable seat back incline (100 degrees from horizontal is optimal)**

- **Changeable seat bottom depth (from the seat back to front edge)**

- **Adjustable seat height**

- **Adjustable seat bottom incline**

- **Seat bottom cushion with firm (dense) foam**

- **Adjustable lumbar support (horizontally and vertically adjustable)**

- **Depth pulsating lumbar support to reduce static load**

- **Adjustable bilateral armrests**

- **Adjustable seat back incline (100-degrees from horizontal is optimal**

- **Adjustable head restraint with lordosis pad**

- **Seat shock absorbers to dampen frequencies between 1- 20 Hz**

- **Linear front-back seat travel to allow differently sized drivers to reach the pedals**

- **Seat back damped to reduce rebounding of the torso in rear-end impacts" (2019a)**

As great as this list looks, it is unlikely to find every one of these features in a single car seat and if it was possible, it would be beyond the budget for many of us. Luckily for us, Hedge used this list to present us with the five most important things we can do when driving a car to reduce the risk of back problems.

Be comfortable. After you have adjusted the seat to suit your body, it should be comfortable to you. If you do not feel comfortable, you will feel it in your back after driving for any length of time. Bounce up and down to test how it will react when driving on the road.

Does the car have all the seat adjustments you would like? If not, you should at least be able to adjust the distance from the pedals and seat height, to accommodate leg length and the backrest angle from 90 degrees and greater. Other great features would be a seat tilt for your legs, adjustable lumbar support, headrest for neck support, and adjustable armrests that are comfortable.

Once you are in the car and driving, change your posture. When it is safe to do so, wiggle and stretch for example when sitting in stationary traffic or waiting at a red light.

Take breaks. Driving is exhausting work, as you have to be on constant alert. To keep mentally alert and to relieve the pressure off your spine, it is good to periodically stop, get out and walk around.

Seat accessories. There are many to choose from: beaded seat backs, wedge cushions, fuzzy covers, etc., whatever adds to your comfort will help reduce the risk of developing back problems (2019a).

Lifting Posture

Not keeping the proper posture while lifting can put unnecessary stress on the muscles, discs, and joints of our lower backs. Muscles can form micro tears, leading to muscle strains, which can be a common cause for back injuries to occur. Improper lifting can cause disc injuries in the lower back, which can lead to back pain, not only in the back but causing sciatica symptoms. Lifting even a light object the wrong way can irritate the joints in your lower back, provoking symptoms (Miller, 2019).

According to Ron Miller, following these three simple steps can prevent back injury while lifting.

- **Bend at the hips while keeping your upper back upright and pointing slightly forward. Most people think bending at the knees prevents back injuries, and while that is better than bending at the waist, it does not ensure that your spine is in the proper position.**

- **Keep your chest forward. When your chest is kept forward and you bend at the hips, your back is kept straight and this should help you avoid spinal injuries. If you bend at the hips and keep your chest out, your knees will automatically bend as well so that the bigger muscles of the legs and hips will bear the weight of the object being lifted. Keeping your chest forward will also help prevent twisting as twisting is another major cause of back injury. Keep your shoulders and hips in line and if you need to change direction, move your hips first and your shoulders will move as well. If you move your shoulders first, twisting will occur and this can lead to a back injury, especially in the joints of the back and pelvis.**

- **Keep the objects being lifted close to your body. More force is required to hold something that is further away from your centre of gravity. This extra force will be placed on your spine, the body's centre of gravity, so holding the object closer to your body will put less stress on your back (2019).**

Sometimes we are not able to bend at the hips to pick up or lift things, so these are three alternative ways to lift things. If you need to pick something small and light off the floor, use what is known as the "Golfer's Lift." This technique consists of lifting one leg up off of the floor and out towards the back to act as a counterbalance for the opposite arm that is going down and forward. If possible, place the other hand on a counter to give even more stability. Although your chest is pointing towards the floor, because your leg is out in the back, it allows the spine to stay straight, avoiding injury. When having to lift something above the level of the waist, use the momentum of the object in your favour. It is basically a controlled movement, where the lifter moves towards the destination of the object while lifting it up and away from the body, requiring less effort. You can also get into a half-kneeling position when having to pick awkward items off of the floor. With this lift, you kneel behind the object with one knee on the floor and the other knee at a 90-degree angle. Now lift the object onto the bended knee and either straighten that knee to propel forward, or the knee that is behind, to help propel backward. While your chest may be pointing downward as you straighten, your spine remains straight, reducing the risk of back injuries. (Ammerman, 2019). Some people may require the aid of a supportive belt to keep proper posture while lifting. If you are carrying something in one arm or on one shoulder, like a purse or bag, switch shoulders/arms frequently. If carrying a backpack, do not lean forward or round your shoulders, distribute the weight evenly, consider using a chest strap.

Sitting Posture

While we know that sitting for long periods of time is not healthy, it cannot be avoided. We all sit throughout the day, some of us are required to sit for extended periods of time, so it is important that we do it properly in order to reduce our risks of injury. According to Stephen Ornstein, this is the proper way to sit:

- Avoid slouching or leaning forward.

- **Arms should be flexed at a 75-90 degree angles at the elbow.**

- **Knees should be even with the hips or slightly higher.**

- **Keep both feet flat on the floor. If both feet cannot be comfortably flat on the floor, a footstool should be used.**

- **Sit with shoulders straight.**

- **Do not sit for too long, get up, walk around and stretch.**

A bad sitting posture can affect your neck and back, particularly your lower lumbar area. Sitting introduces a large amount of pressure on the discs much more than standing, and most chairs and seats actually encourage an unbalanced posture and the flattening of the curve of our lower back causing the head to tilt forward, which also causes poor neck posture. Poor sitting posture will fatigue the back muscles, leading to a poor or slumped posture. Using a back support pillow can help relieve the stress on your back muscles and aid in relieving pressure on discs (Ornstein, n.d.).

To achieve the best sitting posture, the back of your seat should be tilting backward at an angle of 90 to 105 degrees. The back of your knees should not be touching the edge of your chair and the seat should be angled slightly forward to match the natural slope of your lower back. A seat wedge can be used to help adjust the angle of your seat from buttocks to knees (Ornstein, n.d.).

Mattress
A good night's sleep is vital to aiding in the rejuvenation process of the body and mind. Your mattress could not only be impacting the quality of your night's sleep, but it could also be causing you physical pain as well, especially back, shoulder, and hip pain. The general purpose of a mattress is to support

the structures of the spine, including the discs, and muscles to recover from the gravitational and postural strain they undergo throughout the day (Orstein, nd).

There is a correlation between the way you sleep and the firmness of your mattress. If you are a side sleeper or you suffer from hip or shoulder pain, a softer mattress is deemed better for you. Medium for back and side sleepers and firmer for those who sleep on their backs or stomachs. Overall, a medium-firm mattress is the best to go with, especially if you change your positions a lot during the night. General guidelines evolve around the natural shape of the spine and weight should also be considered. Latex and memory foam mix mattresses can be deemed reasonable choice ones to purchase (Orstein, n.d.).

Certain diagnosed back conditions should be an important factor in determining the mattress you purchase and the position in which you sleep.

- **Osteoarthritis.** You should sleep in the fetal position, on your side with your knees curled up. This will open the facet joints and relieve related pressure. Sleeping in a reclining chair or adjustable bed with knees and head elevated can also alleviate pressure and pain.

- **Degenerative disc disease.** To remove pressure on the discs, sleeping on your stomach on a firm mattress is recommended. You can also place a flat pillow under your hips and stomach to further open up the disc space and relieve pressure. If sleeping on your stomach is not desirable, you can sleep on your back with a wedge pillow to elevate your upper spine or use an adjustable bed. Your knees should be slightly bent as well to further relieve pressure on your discs.

- **Spinal Stenosis.** Sleeping in the same position as those with osteoarthritis is recommended, fetal position or in a reclining chair or adjustable bed.

- **Spondylolisthesis.** Pain from spondylolisthesis can best be relieved by sleeping in a reclining chair or mimicking this positioning by placing pillows under the back

- **Herniated lumbar disc.** Depending on the positioning of the disc, you should either sleep on your side or stomach. If it is a foraminal herniated disc, sleeping on your side in the fetal position is best. If you have the most common type, paracentral herniated disc, lying on your stomach may be best.

- **Sleeping in a reclining position is preferable when sleeping with back pain or sciatica.** To test this, if your pain feels worse when you stand up straight and eases when you bend forward, you may get more comfort sleeping in a reclining position. There are several options for sleeping in this position, a reclining chair, an adjustable bed, or a wedge cushion (Staehler, 2017).

Pillows
Pillows do not only support your head while you sleep, when they are used correctly help alleviate and prevent back, neck, shoulder, hip, and other joint pain. Your pillow helps align your upper body, relieving pressure on your spine and alleviating any pressure points. It is important to align the height of your pillow with your sleeping position and your body size. Your neck is curved slightly forward and it is important to keep this curve when you are in a resting position. If your pillow is too high when sleeping on your side or back, it may cause muscle strains on the back of your neck and your shoulders. If your pillow is too low, it will strain the muscles of

your neck. A pillow should maintain a height of four to six inches to give your head, neck, and shoulders (when lying on your back) proper support (Schubbe, 2016).

When choosing a pillow, you need to consider the position you sleep in. If you sleep on your back, you need to choose a pillow that will support the natural curve of your cervical spine while giving adequate support for your head, neck, and shoulders. Your pillow should be flatter than if you were sleeping on your side. Placing another pillow under your knees will also help alleviate back pain by lessening the pressure on your facet joints. Sleeping on one's back seems to be the preferred position for those experiencing acute back pain or recovering from back surgery (Schubbe, 2016).

When sleeping on your side, a thicker pillow is needed to maintain a normal and straight horizontal line while supporting your head and neck. A firm pillow placed between bended knees is also recommended as this will keep the spine in a neutral position. Adding this support between the knees can also alleviate back pain (Schubbe, 2016).

The most stressful sleeping position for your spine is sleeping on your stomach. If you do this, you should use a flat pillow or no pillow at all. If you must sleep in this position as it aids in alleviating your symptoms, it is recommended that you place a flat pillow under your abdomen and pelvis, so that the lower back can be in its natural alignment. If you sleep in multiple positions, you should look for a pillow with high and low sections or a buckwheat hull pillow, that you can easily shape (Schubbe, 2016).

Ergonomics

Ergonomics is the study of the relationship between your work environment and your physical and mental health. Ergonomics can be broken down into two main concentrations, which often overlap. Industrial ergonomics, which is concerned with force and repetition of the task and posture required of the worker. The other is concerned with human factors such as the mental health and wellbeing of the worker. Today, the risk factors of the workplace are divided into three areas: physical characteristics, environmental characteristics, and workplace hazards (Rodts, 2020). While all three of these areas have at least one factor that can cause back injury or pain the first, physical characteristics are tied to back pain with every factor. It is within this area that we will focus.

Computers

Many people today find themselves spending hours in front of a computer, whether it be at work or at home. There are many considerations and determinants to setting up a computer workstation. Hedge recommends considering the following:

How will the computer be used? Will it be used by the same individual or will different people be using it? If used by more than one person, an adjustable arrangement may be necessary. It may not be possible to achieve the best arrangement for everyone, so the extremes may only be met, the shortest and tallest, the thinnest and broadest. How long at a time will the computer station be used? If only for a few minutes at a time, ergonomics may not need to be a priority. If used for more than one hour a day, an ergonomic arrangement should be set up.

What kind of computer will be used? If using a computer for an extended period of time over an hour it is assumed you will be using a desktop system. The keyboard should be separate from the monitor. If not, you should consider buying an external keyboard, preferably a negative tilt, and monitor.

What furniture will you use? Make sure these computer components: mouse, keyboard, and monitor are placed on a stable working station with enough room to be properly arranged. Choose a system that is adjustable, allowing you to tilt the keyboard down away from you, and that allows you to use the mouse as close to your body as possible. This will keep your arms and wrists relaxed.

What chair will be used? If only one person is using the station, choose a comfortable chair, of the correct height, with a good backrest and lumbar support. If more than one person will be using the station, a chair with adjustable height, back, and lumbar support is recommended. The best posture while seated is not the 90 degree upright posture but a reclined position of about 100-110 degrees. Erect sitting puts too much pressure on the spine.

What kind of work will the computer be used for? If the station will be used mainly for word processing, the positioning of the keyboard/mouse is the highest priority. For surfing the net or graphic design, the position of the mouse will be most important. The numeric keyboard/keyboard will be of the highest priority for data entry. If the station will be used mostly for gaming, the positioning of the keyboard/mouse/gamepad will be a top priority.

What can you see? Any paper documents that need to be read should be placed as close to the computer monitor as possible. Use a document holder if you can. This will help prevent excess turning of the neck.

The computer monitor should be placed directly in front of you and whatever you are reading or working on at the time should be at the centre of your screen.

The monitor should be at a comfortable height so that you do not have to tilt your head up or down when viewing the monitor. When seated comfortably the user's eyes should line up with a point about 2-3 inches below the top of the monitor's casing.

If wearing glasses, you should still sit with your back at a 110-degree angle to prevent lower back pain. You may have to tilt your monitor back at an angle and adjust the height to be able to see the screen without tilting your head back or craning your neck forward. The centre of the computer monitor should be about 17.5 degrees below eye level.

To maintain a comfortable viewing distance from your monitor, you should be able to sit comfortably and your monitor should be at an arm's length away from you. At this distance, you should be able to see the entirety of the screen without having to move your neck. If you cannot, adjust your font size or the screen's magnifying imaging instead of moving the monitor closer to you.

Make sure you are using a good quality screen and the resolution is sharp and the right size. This can be adjusted to personal preferences on any quality screen.

Eye check-ups are important for anyone but especially those over 50, who work with visual technology every day. If you cannot seem to get the resolution right, you may need an eye check-up.

Posture. Good posture is the best way to avoid a computer work related back injury. You should be able to reach the keyboard keys with your wrists flat and straight—not bent up or down or left or right. The angle of your elbow should be 90 degrees or greater to avoid nerve compression at the elbows giving tingling into the hands. When using the mouse, your upper arm and elbow should be as close to the body as possible and your wrist should be straight. Be sure to not overreach when using the mouse. Sit back in your chair and use a comfortable back support. Feet placed firmly on the floor or on a footrest. Your head and neck should be as straight as possible and you should feel relaxed.

Keep things close. Things that are used frequently should be placed close by to prevent over-stretching when reaching for them, such as for a phone or stapler.

A good ergonomic workstation arrangement. For the general computer user, they should be able to work in a neutral, relaxed, ideal typing posture to minimise any risk of injury. The keyboard should be on a height-adjustable negative tilt surface. The mouse should be on a flat surface closer to your body and your wrist should be flat while browsing the internet.

Where will the computer be used? This last question may indirectly lead you to sit with a poor posture or to move in ways that may lead to injury, so these considerations may seem less important but they can still save you from injury if addressed properly. Make sure the lighting is not too bright or causes a glare off your screen. If you do you may have to adjust your screens brightness or get an anti-glare screen to go over your monitor. Do not move your monitor out of the light, so that you have to curve your neck to see it. If you move your monitor, you have to move everything else to keep your station ergonomical. Make sure your computer is placed somewhere with proper ventilation and adequate heating and cooling so that you can remain relaxed. Noise can cause you to tense your muscles and thus be a factor for causing injury. Try to work in a quiet location or use low, soft music to drown out noises.

Chapter 6: Spinal Injections and Surgery

Some people require more invasive treatments such as surgeries and injections to deal with their back pain. There are two types of spinal surgeries: open/ traditional surgery or minimally invasive surgery.

Lumbar Epidural

A lumbar epidural steroid injection (ESIs) consists of a mixture of anaesthetic and steroid medication being injected directly into the epidural space around the spinal cord and nerve roots. ESIs are a very common treatment for lower back and leg pain that has been around for decades. ESIs are given to reduce inflammation around the nerve endings to reduce pain and to improve mobility of the lower back and legs so that the patient can be more engaged in Manual therapy exercises and rehabilitation programs. Typically, ESIs are used to treat herniated discs, degenerative disc disease, and spinal stenosis, when these conditions exist in the lumbar region of the spine. ESIs are a step once the use of medications and Manual therapy has been proven unsuccessful and before surgery is considered (Staehler, 2020).

Epidural steroid injections are most effective during episodes of acute back or leg pain. The relief they give is only temporary, normally estimated at anywhere from one week to one year. Sometimes they are not effective at all. If effective the following are some of the benefits for the recipient: reduction of nerve inflammation and pain, may now be able to readily participate more in Manual therapy exercises without experiencing pain, and you may experience enough pain relief that surgery can be postponed or even cancelled. According to Staehler, "with 70% to 90% of patients experiencing pain relief from these injections, lasting from a week to a year...up to 3 injections may be administered over a 12 month period" (2020).

Selective Nerve Root Block (SNRB)

Selective Nerve Root Block (SNRB) injections can be just an anaesthetic or an anaesthetic and steroid mixture used to treat or diagnose an inflamed spinal nerve. Pain signals from the treated nerve may be reduced by inhibiting the actions of certain enzymes that cause irritation and pain, blocking certain fibres within the nerve that transmit pain to the brain and thus reducing pain transmission. (Funiciello, 2019).

Facet Joint Injection
The facet joints of the spine may become painful due to arthritis, injury, or mechanical stress which may be treated with a facet joint injection. These injections consist of an anaesthetic or an anaesthetic and steroid (cortisone) mixture being injected into the joints to reduce inflammation.

Sacroiliac Injections
Sacroiliac injections can potentially be administered to a patient if prescribed medication and Manual therapy do not aid in relieving the pain associated with sacroiliac joint pain. The injections for sacroiliac joint pain are the same as the Medical Practitioner would have given to diagnose the condition; a mixture of anaesthetic and steroid. The relief from this injection will usually start working in three to seven days. The benefit of these injections is that you should be able to move more freely without much pain allowing you to participate more efficiently in Manual therapy. If the pain returns, your Medical Practitioner may consider repeating these injections every two to four-months. But if no relief is experienced over a period of seven days. Your Medical Practitioner may recommend referring you for a surgical opinion (Wheeler, 2019).

Prolotherapy
Prolotherapy kickstarts the body's natural immune system by injecting an irritant into the soft tissue of an injured joint. The body will start to strengthen and repair the damaged soft tissue commonly being ligaments. As the ligament strengthens, the joint will stabilise, easing the pain or even making it disappear. Medical Practitioners commonly use these injections to treat injured joints and ligaments of the back, they can also be used to treat knees, hips, and shoulder symptoms. Those with degenerative disc disease and arthritis may also wish to enquire about receiving prolotherapy injections to help relieve pain. During an injection session. The benefits of prolotherapy are clear in that it is an all-natural permanent treatment that can not only relieve pain but also strengthen, stabilise and improve the overall function of the back and joints (Fletcher, 2019).

Trigger Point Injections
Trigger point injections (TPIs) are used to treat muscles that do not relax and become knotted forming trigger points. These muscles can often irritate the nerves around them, causing pain in other parts of the body. The needle injected into the trigger point may contain an anaesthetic or saline, it may also include an anti-inflammatory such as a steroid. The injection alleviates pain by making the trigger point inactive thus giving patients pain relief (Wheeler, 2020).

Platelet Rich Plasma
Platelet-rich plasma (PRP) injections are believed to trigger your body to grow new healthy cells and promote healing. The plasma in your blood contains protein that supports cell growth. By isolating plasma from blood, researchers have been able to produce concentrated PRP, which they believe will promote faster healing. It is this concentrated PRP that is injected into the injured area. Many famous athletes have been using PRP injections to speed up the healing of injuries. Where PRP injections have been

approved, Medical Practitioners have used them to treat, tendon injuries, acute injuries, osteoarthritis, and post-surgical repair. The treatment involves drawing blood out of the patient, then placing the blood sample into a centrifuge. The blood is then spun, causing the components to separate, with this separated plasma then being injected into the injured area of the patient. This meaning you are getting back a plasma concentrate from your own blood (Nall, 2018).

Surgeries

There are two types of spinal surgeries: open/ conventional surgeries and keyhole/minimal/minimal access spine surgery. Compressed discs and tumours can be treated through keyhole surgeries. These surgeries have many advantages, such as less blood loss, less damage to neighbouring tissues, and reduced healing time but they also require special training and specialised equipment (Keyhole Spine Surgery, 2017).

Spinal Decompression Surgery

If spinal decompression therapy IDD doesn't work, your Medical Practitioner may suggest spinal decompression surgery. This is usually a last resort to deal with bulging or ruptured discs, bony growths, or other spinal problems. The surgery may relieve pain, numbness, tingling or weakness caused by pressure exerted on the spinal cord or nerves. There are different types of spinal decompression surgery your Medical Practitioner may suggest. Besides laminectomy, which will be discussed later, there is also discectomy where a portion of the disc is removed, foraminotomy where a bone or other tissue is removed, osteophyte removal, bony growths, or corpectomy which involves removing a vertebral body with discs between the vertebrae. Risks associated with spinal decompression surgery are infection, bleeding, blood clots, nerve and tissue damage. Unfortunately, it is not a given that patients will benefit from this surgery (Wheeler, 2019a).

Spinal Fusion Surgery

Spinal fusion surgery is when extra bone is used to permanently join two or more vertebrae together so that no space remains. While spinal fusion surgery affects flexibility, it is useful for conditions that cause pain through movement including but not limited to, tumours, spinal stenosis, herniated discs, degenerative disc disease, etc. A discectomy is sometimes necessary during spinal fusion surgery. This involves removing a diseased disc and replacing it with bone grafts to maintain the right height. The Medical Practitioner will then fuse the two vertebrae on either side of the removed disc to create stability (Giorgi, 2019).

The post-surgery period after a spinal fusion surgery can range from taking three to six months on average. Since your flexibility is limited post surgery, you may have to learn a new way to walk, sit, and stand. You may have to wear a brace to keep your spine properly aligned and attend frequent physical rehabilitation sessions. The areas above and below the fusion may cause pain over time as they will now take more strain to compensate for the lack of movement at the fused segment (Giorgi, 2019).

Laminectomy

Laminectomy is the removal of the lamina, or the vertebral arch of the spine, and any bone spurs to reduce pressure on the spinal cord. Pressure on the spinal cord or nerve roots can cause back pain, leg numbness or weakness and difficulty walking. A laminectomy is most commonly performed on patients who have spinal stenosis and their symptoms interfering with everyday activities. During a laminectomy, the Medical Practitioner may also need to perform a spinal fusion and/or a foraminotomy, which is the widening of the area where the nerve roots pass through the spine thus reliving patients of their symptoms (Phillips, 2017).

Keyhole Lumbar Discectomy

Keyhole lumbar discectomy is a more advanced form of discectomy which is much less invasive than conventional open surgery. Through the use of advanced technology, this minimally invasive spine surgery (MISS) results in minimal damage to normal tissues and reduced post-surgery recovery time. Tubal retractors are inserted into very small incisions, right into the spinal column creating a tunnel to the area that needs to be operated on. This tube holds back the sounding muscles from the area being operated on, minimalizing the risk of blood loss, and damage to muscles, ligaments, and bones that can occur with more traditional open surgeries. This type of keyhole surgery is most commonly used for herniated lumbar discs (KeyHole Spine Surgery, 2017).

Lumbar Disc Replacement

Lumbar disc replacement is an alternative to spinal fusion surgery and consists of replacing a worn or degenerated disc in your lower back with an artificial disc made of metal or a combination of metal and plastic. Lumbar disc replacement may be an option if you have not had other spinal surgeries, your pain comes from only one or two discs in your lower back, you have no joint disease or compression on your nerves in your lower back, you are not excessively overweight, and you have no spine deformities. A lumbar disc replacement is a riskier surgery than a spinal fusion surgery due to it requiring greater access to the spine. Potential side effects are infection, dislocation or failure of the implant, losing or problems with the positioning of the implant, narrowing and stiffening of the spine (Lumbar Disc Replacement, n.d.).

Conclusion

There are several things you can do to reduce or prevent your back pain from worsening. Changing a few daily habits can help you relieve pressure, reduce strain, strengthen your muscles and protect your spine, allowing you to maintain a healthier more pain-free back. Dr. William Morrison suggests we adopt the following ten daily habits to stop back pain:

- **Use a pillow.** Sleep with a pillow under your knees if you sleep on your back or between your knees if you sleep on your side. This will help keep your spine in its natural alignment and relieve pressure.

- **Work your core.** It is important that you have strong back and abdomen muscles that are able to support your spine without experiencing muscle strains or spasms. You should work on your core muscles as part of your exercise routine at least twice a week.

- **Calcium and vitamin D.** Increase your calcium and vitamin D intake to help strengthen your bones. Osteoporosis is a common cause of back pain in the elder population so keeping bones healthy is important throughout your life. Calcium can be found in milk, yogurt, and leafy greens. Fatty fish, egg yolks, beef liver, and cheese all contain vitamin D.

- **Change your footwear.** Wear comfortable low heeled shoes so that you will not be straining your back while standing. Less than a one inch heel is best for your back.

- **Straighten up.** Bad posture puts unnecessary strain and stress on your back, while good posture aids in protecting the components of your spine.

Don't round your shoulders, slouch or bend sideways while standing.

- **Don't slump over your desk. Sitting posture is just as important as standing posture and sitting incorrectly can put added unnecessary pressure on your spine. If you are sitting for an extended period, make sure your chair is comfortable, provides back support and your knees are slightly above your hips, with your feet planted firmly on the floor.**

- **Mingle. Whether at a business function or a social gathering, don't spend an extended time sitting or standing in one place. Get up and move!**

- **Refrain from smoking. Nicotine restricts blood flow to the discs in the spine which can aid in making them dry out and crack or rupture predisposing you to disc issues. Smoking also reduces the amount of oxygen in the blood and oxygen, reducing the nutrients available to the soft tissues of the back. This makes the smoker more vulnerable to back pain and injury than the non smoker.**

- **Lighten your load. Improper lifting can damage your back, whether it is done repetitively or occasionally. It can be something as simple as a handbag, laptop bag, or briefcase that causes the injury. Whenever possible, take some of that weight off your shoulders, by carrying less, switching sides, distributing the weight, or using a rolling cart.**

- **Stretch. Keep moving to keep the circulation going in your back. Sitting, standing, or lying down for too long is not healthy for your back. Get up, walk around, and stretch multiple times throughout the day!**

Real life case studies of treatment approaches performed on patients

Case 1 the use of IDD therapy

Patient X was a 47 year old male predominantly desk based who worked as an accountant

They suffered from an episode of lower back pain after bending forward to do their shoelaces and suddenly felt a sharp pain in the lower back.

Tried a course of 5 sessions of manual therapy, had acupuncture, dry cupping and tried to do exercise's for their lower back but all with minimal relief.

Was referred for a MRI scan to the lower back and it was revealed that they had a "protruding disc bulge at....." add image as well of scan

A course of IDD was recommended for the patients symptoms as it was a disc bulge and the aim of using the IDD was to help with traction long the spine and taking pressure off of the discs.

Case 2 the use of shockwave for muscle knots

Patient Y was a 30 year old women who was desk based and very active, training to become yoga teacher.

On examination and through palpation it was diagnosed that her issues in her shoulders were muscle knots and tension built up from over straining in a yoga pose and also a build up of tension in the trapezius muscle.

A course of three shockwave sessions was done once a week on the muscle knots in her trapezius muscle and she felt a lot of relief from this.

Case study 3 the use of acupuncture

Patient W was a patient who was 50 years old, works very long hours over 16 hours a day at his desk in a high pressured and highly stressful environment

He developed lower back pain and had an MRI scan that noted disc degeneration. On consultation it was decided that a course of IDD would be the best course of treatment for the patients symptoms as the IDD would aid in adding a light pumping action in the lower back and get blood into the disc to help with the degeneration

It was noted on standing examination that the patient had a very acute rotation in his back since his back pain started.

We did some acupuncture into the muscles of the lower back primarily the lumbar erector spinae to help the muscles relax as performing acupuncture on to spasming muscles that are spasming to protect the lower back when there is any back problems would help with the IDD to be more effective as the muscles would be less tight and the IDD machine could target and perform traction more readily.

From doing the acupuncture on the patients lower back the muscle relaxed and he was able to sleep much better after each acupuncture session and the IDD therapy was more effective in treating his back symptoms.

Case study 4 the use of dry cupping and massage

Patient Z was a..... who presented with neck and shoulder pain after sleeping awkwardly they felt.

It was diagnosed that the stiff neck was in relation to the joints in the neck the facets being locked from sleeping in an awkward portion, this thus caused the muscles in the neck and shoulder region to become stiff and take up a guarding nature to protect the neck

the patient lost a lot of mobility in their neck and felt knots in the shoulders.

It was decided to do some dry cupping and massage in the neck and shoulder muscles primarily targeting the rhomboid muscles in the shoulder blade

, after 1 session the patient felt a lot of relief.

The reason for picking to do massage and dry cupping into the neck and shoulder blade muscles is because when muscles waste guarded massage can help with the circulation and aid in getting fresh blood and nutrients to the muscles to help them repair as blood is what carries nutrients around the body, the aim of the dry cupping was to get rid of the old blood with the use of the suction and attract the new blood to the area in this instance the muscles.

Author Biography
Matthew Irvine is an experienced Osteopathic Physician working in the UK in private practice. Since he was young he had high ambitions to help as many patients as he could overcome their often stubborn and debilitating pain. With Matthew's extensive experience and expertise, he has decided to create this book to help guide patients in better understanding and finding solutions to dealing with their back pain.

Acknowledgements

I would like to thanks all my friends and family who help me everyday to be the best version of myself and who give me strength and courage which is needed in plenty when writing a book. Thank you to my wonderful family for helping me to learn about the wonders of Osteopathy and introducing me to a profession where I get to help and meet so many great people. To my dearest little brother every decision I do and make is for you to give you the best life. I hope I make you proud.

QR codes with links to reviews and testimonials of clients after different techniques used on them to help with their back issues

Before and after an MRI scan of a clients disc

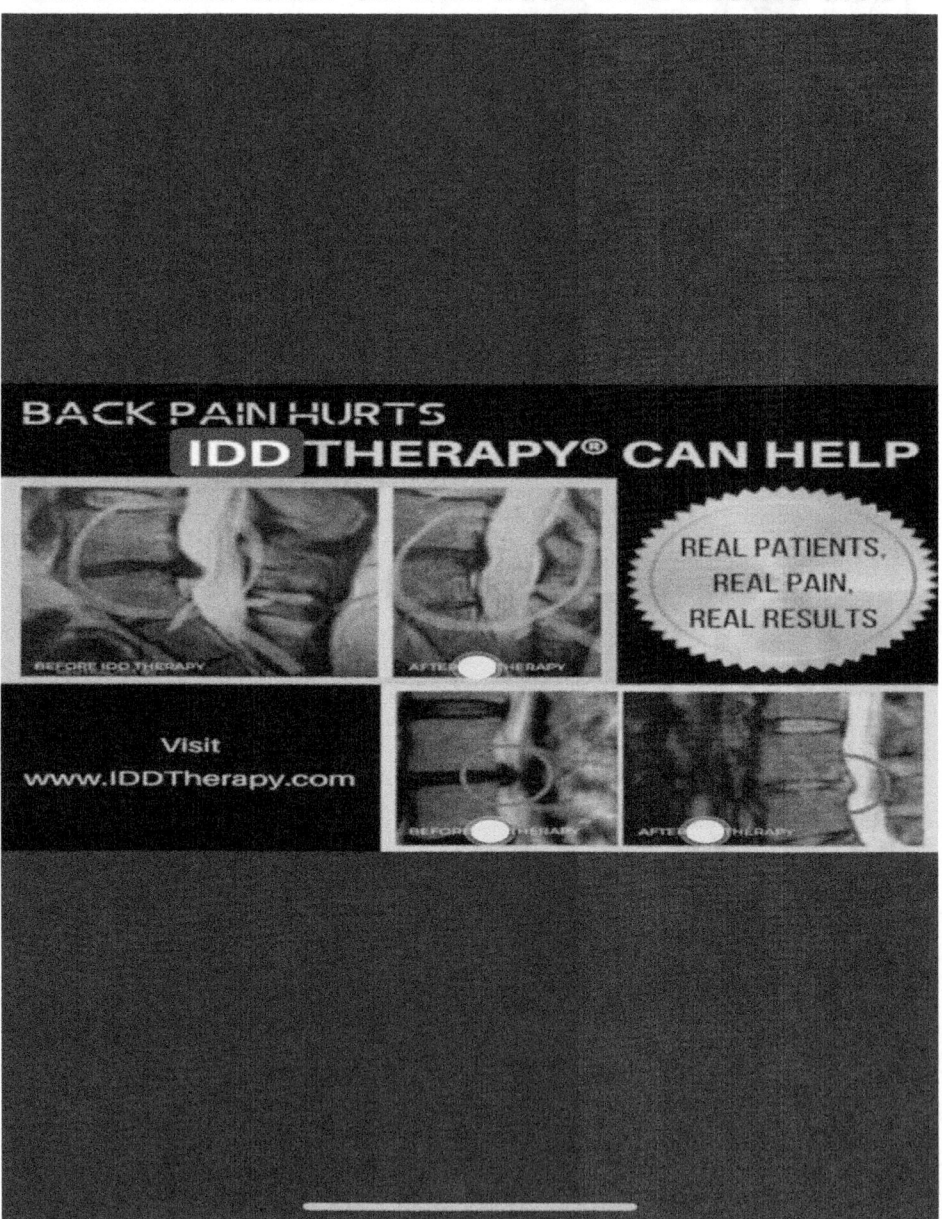

issue

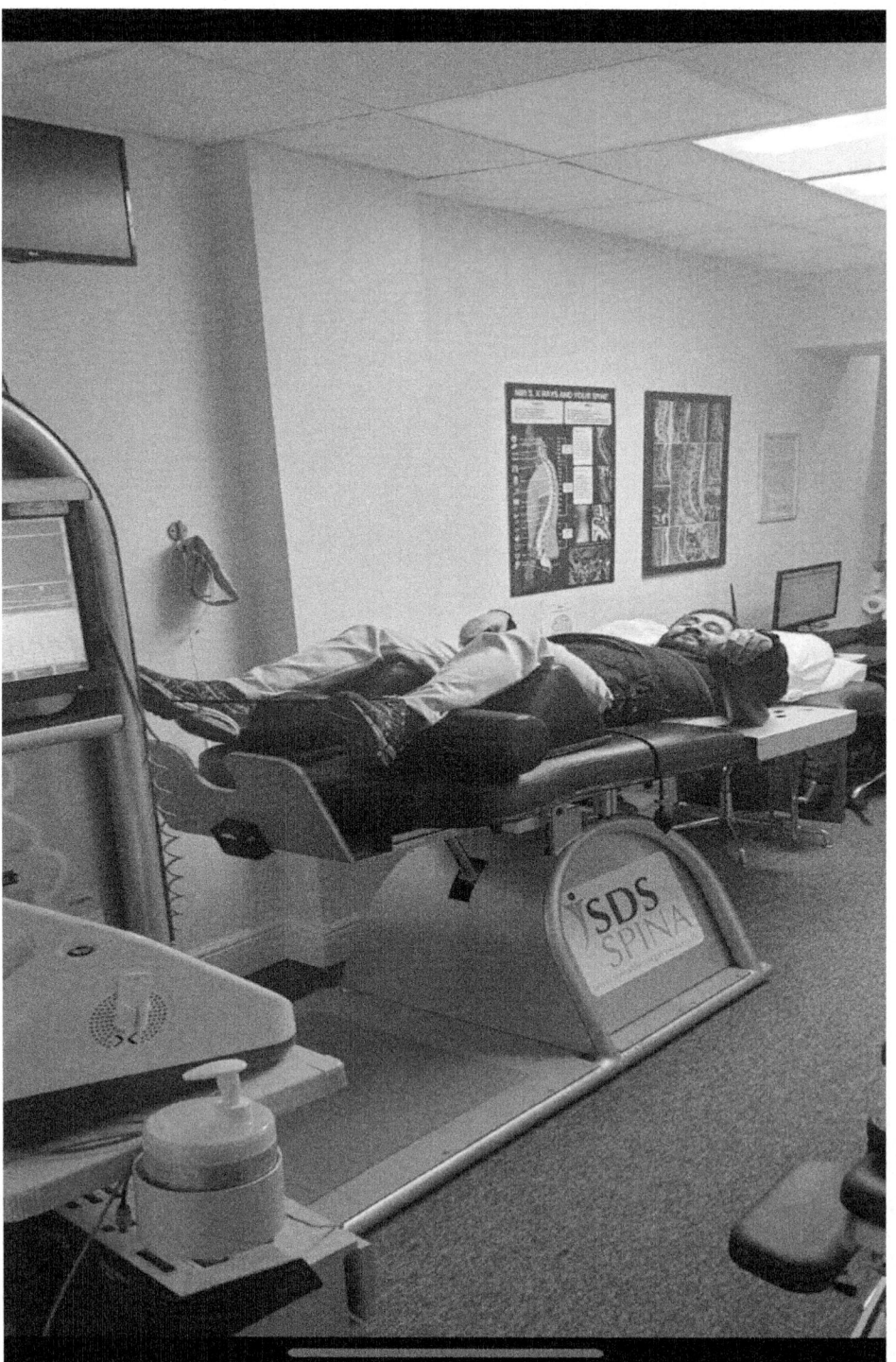

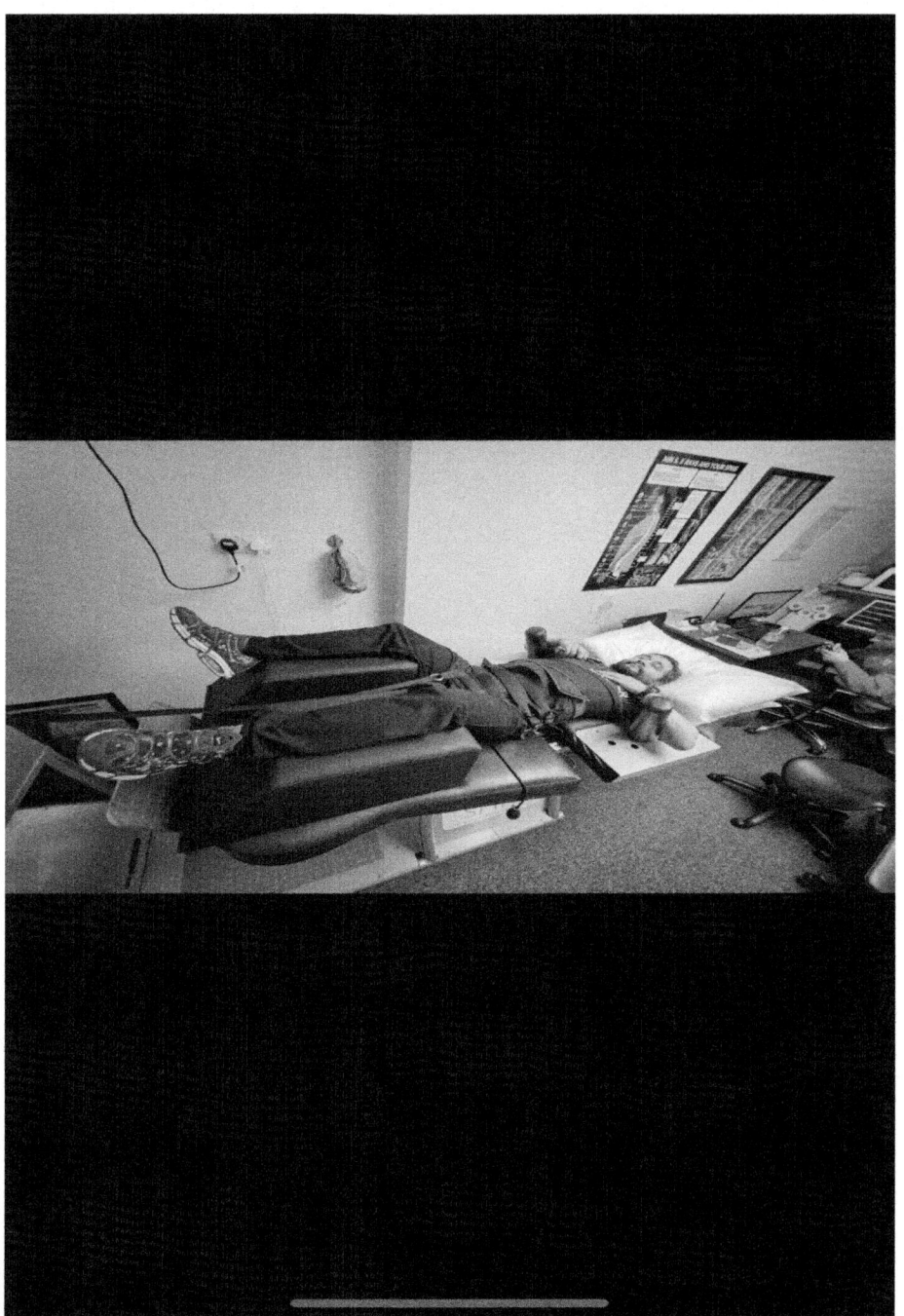

References

Afshar, M. (2017, December 4). What is shockwave therapy? | Lifemark. Lifemark.ca. https://www.lifemark.ca/blog-post/what-shockwave-therapy

Ammerman, J. (2019, August 12). Is Your Cell Phone Killing Your Back? SpineUniverse. https://www.spineuniverse.com/wellness/ergonomics/your-cell-phone-killing-your-back

Asher, A. (2020, January 6). How to Get out of Bed Without a Backache. Verywell Health. https://www.verywellhealth.com/protect-back-when-getting-out-of-bed-tips-296441

Baker, R. (2013, March 22). Cervical, Thoracic and Lumbar Facet Joint Injections. Spine-Health. https://www.spine-health.com/treatment/injections/cervical-thoracic-and-lumbar-facet-joint-injections

Ben-Yishay, A. (2012, April 25). Lumbar Radiculopathy. Spine-Health. https://www.spine-health.com/conditions/lower-back-pain/lumbar-radiculopathy

Burke, D. (2018, August 7). Human Leukocyte Antigen B27 (HLA-B27). Healthline. https://www.healthline.com/health/hla-b27-antigen

Busch, F. (2019). How Yoga Helps the Back. Spine-Health. https://www.spine-health.com/wellness/yoga-pilates-tai-chi/how-yoga-helps-back

Connor, E. (2018, September 17). Nerve Conduction Velocity: Purpose, Procedure & Results. Healthline. https://www.healthline.com/health/nerve-conduction-velocity#preparation

Cronkleton, E. (2020, May 29). Posture Exercises: 12 Exercises to Improve Your Posture. Healthline. https://www.healthline.com/health/posture-exercises

Cupping: Back Pain, Neck Pain, Types, Benefits, Treatment. (2020, August 19). Cleveland Clinic.

https://my.clevelandclinic.org/health/treatments/16554-cupping

Diagnosing Muscle and Bone Disorders With CT Scans. (2019, June 6). Envision Radiology. https://www.envrad.com/diagnosing-muscle-and-bone-disorders-with-ct-scans/#:~:text=Doctors%20can%20look%20at%20CT

Dreyfuss, P. (2019, February 5). SI Joint Injection Information. SpineUniverse. https://www.spineuniverse.com/conditions/sacroiliac-joint-dysfunction/sacroiliac-joint-injection-information

Electrodiagnostics | What a Patient Should Expect. (n.d.). Https://Www.treatingpain.com/. Retrieved March 18, 2021, from https://www.treatingpain.com/treatments/electrodiagnostics/

Fletcher, J. (2017, December 17). Prolotherapy: Uses, side effects, and costs. Www.medicalnewstoday.com. https://www.medicalnewstoday.com/articles/320330#benefits

Forcum, T., & Hyde, T. (2004, May 24). Techniques for Effective Exercise Walking. Spine-Health. https://www.spine-health.com/wellness/exercise/techniques-effective-exercise-walking

Funiciello, M. (2019, June 6). Selective Nerve Root Block Injections. Spine-Health. https://www.spine-health.com/treatment/injections/selective-nerve-root-block-injections

Garland, A. (2017, January 4). Single Photon Emission Computed Tomography (SPECT). News-Medical.net. https://www.news-medical.net/life-sciences/Single-Photon-Emission-Computed-Tomography-(SPECT).aspx

Giorgi, A. (2019, March 5). Spinal Fusion Surgery: Uses, Procedure, and Recovery. Healthline. https://www.healthline.com/health/spinal-fusion

Glosten, B. (2003, March 21). Pilates Exercise and Back Pain. Spine-Health. https://www.spine-health.com/wellness/yoga-pilates-tai-chi/pilates-exercise-and-back-pain

Gordon, S. (2020, May 5). The Buzz on TENS Units for Back Pain. SpineUniverse. https://www.spineuniverse.com/treatments/buzz-tens-units-back-pain

Hasz, M. (2015, September 15). Sacroiliac Joint Pain and Inflammation. Arthritis-Health. https://www.arthritis-health.com/types/general/sacroiliac-joint-pain-and-inflammation

Hazlegreaves, S. (2019, November 11). How can IDD Therapy help unresolved back pain and sciatica? Open Access Government. https://www.openaccessgovernment.org/idd-therapy-back-pain-and-sciatica/77448/

Hecht, M. (2019, February 15). The DEXA Scan Bone Density Test: Preparation, Procedure, Results. Healthline. https://www.healthline.com/health/dexa-scan

Hedge, A. (2019a, March 1). Driving and Back Care. SpineUniverse. https://www.spineuniverse.com/wellness/ergonomics/driving-back-care

Hedge, A. (2019b, September 17). Ergonomic Guidelines for Computer Workstations - 10 Steps for Users. SpineUniverse. https://www.spineuniverse.com/wellness/ergonomics/ergonomic-guidelines-computer-workstations-10

Hochschuler, S. (2004, August 4). How Exercise Helps the Back. Spine-Health. https://www.spine-health.com/wellness/exercise/how-exercise-helps-back

Humphreys, R. (2004, February 19). Tai Chi for Posture and Back Pain. Spine-Health. https://www.spine-health.com/wellness/yoga-pilates-tai-chi/tai-chi-posture-and-back-pain

Key Hole Spine Surgery: Making Spine Surgery Easier. (2017, July 28). Aster Medcity. https://astermedcity.com/blog/readmore/key-hole-spine-surgery-making-spine-surgery

Krans, B. (2018, September 29). Bone Scan. Healthline; Healthline Media. https://www.healthline.com/health/bone-scan

Laguipo, A. (2019, January 8). How Does Infrared Therapy Work? News-Medical.net. https://www.news-medical.net/health/How-Does-Infrared-Therapy-Work.aspx

Locked facet joints are easy to diagnose and treat. (2017, June 6). Sperling Medical Group. http://sperlingmedicalgroup.com/locked-facet-joints-are-easy-to-diagnose-and-treat/

Low back pain - acute: MedlinePlus Medical Encyclopedia. (2018). Medlineplus.gov. https://medlineplus.gov/ency/article/007425.htm

Low Back Strain and Sprain – Symptoms, Diagnosis and Treatments. (n.d.). Www.aans.org. Retrieved March 7, 2021, from https://www.aans.org/Patients/Neurosurgical-Conditions-and-Treatments/Low-Back-Strain-and-Sprain#:~:text=Lumbar%20muscle%20strain%20is%20caused

Lumbar Disk Replacement. (n.d.). Www.hopkinsmedicine.org. Retrieved March 19, 2021, from https://www.hopkinsmedicine.org/health/treatment-tests-and-therapies/lumbar-disk-

replacement#:~:text=Lumbar%20disk%20repla
cement%20involves%20replacing

Lumbar Spinal Stenosis. (2020).
https://www.hopkinsmedicine.org/health/cond
itions-and-diseases/lumbar-spinal-stenosis

Malanga, G. (2019, March 14). Sitting Disease
and Its Impact on Your Spine. SpineUniverse.
https://www.spineuniverse.com/wellness/ergo
nomics/sitting-disease-its-impact-your-spine

Malanga, G., & MD. (2019, February 19). Ice
and Heat Treats Back Pain. SpineUniverse.
https://www.spineuniverse.com/treatments/ph
ysical-therapy/physical-therapy-tens-
ultrasound-heat-cryotherapy

Mary Anne Dunkin. (2010, January 14). Back
Pain in Pregnancy. WebMD; WebMD.
https://www.webmd.com/baby/guide/back-
pain-in-pregnancy#1

McIntosh, J. (2071, February 23). Back pain:
Causes, symptoms, and treatments.
Www.medicalnewstoday.com.
https://www.medicalnewstoday.com/articles/1
72943

Meyler, Z. (2020, May 26). Getting an
Accurate Back Pain Diagnosis. Spine-Health.
https://www.spine-
health.com/treatment/diagnostic-
tests/getting-accurate-back-pain-diagnosis

Miller, R. (2019). Avoid Back Injury with the
Right Lifting Techniques. Spine-Health.
https://www.spine-
health.com/conditions/sports-and-spine-
injuries/avoid-back-injury-right-lifting-
techniques

Minx, E. (2020, April 24). Activator Method
Chiropractic Technique. Spine-Health.
https://www.spine-
health.com/treatment/chiropractic/activator-
method-chiropractic-technique

Mitchell, E. (2019, August 13). Back pain and doing daily chores. Www.bupa.co.uk. https://www.bupa.co.uk/newsroom/ourviews/daily-chores-back-pain

Moore, K. (2018, September 29). Spondylolisthesis: Symptoms, Causes, and Treatment. Healthline. https://www.healthline.com/health/spondylolisthesis#causes

Morris, R. (2015, February 9). What Is Spinal Manipulation? Healthline; Healthline Media. https://www.healthline.com/health/back-pain/spinal-manipulation

Morrison, W. (2017, December 14). 10 Daily Habits To Stop Back Pain. Healthline. https://www.healthline.com/health/back-pain-management

Mueller, B. (2002, May 10). Massage Therapy for Lower Back Pain. Spine-Health. https://www.spine-health.com/wellness/massage-therapy/massage-therapy-lower-back-pain#:~:text=Benefits%20of%20Massage%20Therapy&text=Massage%20improves%20blood%20circulation%2C%20which

Nall, R. (2018, September 3). What Is PRP? Healthline; Healthline Media. https://www.healthline.com/health/prp

Nall, R. (2019a, March 22). Lower Left Back Pain: Causes, Treatments, and When to Be Worried. Healthline. https://www.healthline.com/health/fitness-exercise/fixing-common-source-lower-back-pain

Nall, R. (2019b, November 12). Spinal cord: Anatomy, functions, and injuries. Www.medicalnewstoday.com. https://www.medicalnewstoday.com/articles/326984

Nava, A. (n.d.). 7 Ways to Treat Chronic Back Pain Without Surgery. Www.hopkinsmedicine.org. Retrieved March 7, 2021, from https://www.hopkinsmedicine.org/health/cond itions-and-diseases/back-pain/7-ways-to-treat-chronic-back-pain-without-surgery#:~:text=Chronic%20back%20pain%20i s%20usually

Nazir, S. (2018, July 17). Cupping for Chronic Back and Lower Back Pain. Www.practo.com. https://www.practo.com/healthfeed/cupping-for-chronic-back-and-lower-back-pain-34078/post

Ornstein, S. (n.d.). Back Support Belts - Benefits & Types Of Supports For Back Pain. Neck Solutions. Retrieved March 19, 2021, from https://www.necksolutions.com/back-support-belts/

Phillips, N. (2017, July 8). Laminectomy: Purpose, Procedure, and Risks. Healthline. https://www.healthline.com/health/laminectom y

Pressman, P. (2020, September 23). Everything You Need to Know About a Spinal Tap. Verywell Health. https://www.verywellhealth.com/lumbar-punctures-common-questions-answered-2488675

Revord, J. (2012, September 14). What Is Piriformis Syndrome? Spine-Health. https://www.spine-health.com/conditions/sciatica/what-piriformis-syndrome
Richeimer, S., MD, & Spinasanta, S. (2019, February 4). Spine Muscles in Pain? Myofascial Pain Syndrome May Be to Blame. SpineUniverse. https://www.spineuniverse.com/conditions/ch ronic-pain/spine-muscles-pain-myofascial-pain-syndrome-may-blame

Rodts, M. (2020, February 3). Ergonomics: The Human Body and Injury Prevention. SpineUniverse. https://www.spineuniverse.com/wellness/ergonomics/ergonomics-human-body-injury-prevention

Schubbe, J. (2004, May 17). Good Posture Helps Reduce Back Pain. Spine-Health. https://www.spine-health.com/wellness/ergonomics/good-posture-helps-reduce-back-pain

Schubbe, J. (2016, March 30). Pillow Support and Comfort. Spine-Health. https://www.spine-health.com/wellness/sleep/pillow-support-and-comfort

Services, D. of H. & H. (2020, March). Back pain – disc problems. Www.betterhealth.vic.gov.au. https://www.betterhealth.vic.gov.au/health/conditionsandtreatments/back-pain-disc-problems#:~:text=Symptoms%20of%20disc%20Oproblems

Shiel, W. (2020, March 10). What Is a Lumbar Discography Procedure? MedicineNet. https://www.medicinenet.com/what_is_a_lumbar_discography_procedure/article.htm

Silver, N. (2019, March 11). Pinched Nerve in Lower Back: Causes, Symptoms, and Treatments. Healthline. https://www.healthline.com/health/back-pain/pinched-nerve-in-lower-back

Spinal Arthritis (Arthritis in the Back or Neck). (n.d.). Www.hopkinsmedicine.org. https://www.hopkinsmedicine.org/health/conditions-and-diseases/spinal-arthritis

Spinasanta, S., Harrop, J. S., MD, & FACS. (2019, August 6). Ultrasonography is Ultrasound Imaging Used to Help Diagnose Spinal Disorders. SpineUniverse. https://www.spineuniverse.com/exams-tests/ultrasonography-ultrasound-imaging-used-help-diagnose-spinal-disorders#:~:text=Though%20more%20resear ch%20needs%20to

Spine Structure & Function | Cleveland Clinic. (2015). Cleveland Clinic. https://my.clevelandclinic.org/health/articles/1 0040-spine-structure-and-function

Staehler, R. (2017, October 25). Mattresses and Sleep Positions for Each Back Pain Diagnosis. Spine-Health. https://www.spine-health.com/wellness/sleep/mattresses-and-sleep-positions-each-back-pain-diagnosis

Staehler, R. (2020, October 22). Lumbar Epidural Steroid Injections for Low Back Pain and Sciatica. Spine-Health. https://www.spine-health.com/treatment/injections/lumbar-epidural-steroid-injections-low-back-pain-and-sciatica

Stanborough, R. (2019, March 20). What is Kinesiology Tape? Healthline; Healthline Media. https://www.healthline.com/health/kinesiology -tape

Wheeler, T. (2019a, May 17). Spinal Decompression Therapy. WebMD. https://www.webmd.com/back-pain/guide/spinal-decompression-therapy-surgical-nonsurgical

Wheeler, T. (2019b, December 11). Treatments for Your Sacroiliac Joint Pain. WebMD. https://www.webmd.com/back-pain/si-joint-dysfunction-treatment

Wheeler, T. (2020, March 15). Trigger Point Injection (TPI) for Pain Management. WebMD. https://www.webmd.com/pain-management/guide/trigger-point-injection

White, A. (2017, October 6). Acupuncture for Back Pain: Does it Work? Healthline. https://www.healthline.com/health/acupunctur e-for-back-pain

Printed in Dunstable, United Kingdom